D0446148

WALTER GRETZKY

On Family, Hockey and Healing

National Spokesperson for the
Heart and Stroke Foundation of Canada

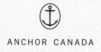

ANCHOR CANADA

Anchor Canada and colophon are trademarks.

National Library of Canada Cataloguing in Publication

Gretzky, Walter
On family, hockey and healing / Walter Gretzky.

ISBN 0-385-65941-5

1. Gretzky, Walter. 2. Gretzky, Wayne, 1961– Family.
3. Cerebrovascular disease—Patients—Canada—Biography. I. Title.

RC388.5.G74 2002   796.962'092   C2002-902930-9

Photographs from Wayne Gretzky's marriage to Janet Jones, by Garneau Studios, appear courtesy of the Gretzky family. Photograph of Walter Gretzky on the golf course, by Brian Thompson, *Brantford Expositor*, appears courtesy of Stephan, Sylvie, Paul and Daniel Namisniak. Photograph of Wayne Gretzky receiving the Order of Canada, by Sgt. Christian Coulombe, Rideau Hall, appears courtesy of the Gretzky family. All other text photographs appear courtesy of Walter Gretzky and his family.

Cover photograph: Curtis Lantinga
Cover design: CS Richardson
Printed and bound in Canada

Published in Canada by
Anchor Canada, a division of
Random House of Canada Limited

Visit Random House of Canada Limited's website: www.randomhouse.ca

TRANS   10 9 8 7 6 5 4 3 2 1

To my grandchildren:
Paulina
Ty
Trevor
Tristan
Nathan
Austin
Zachery
Kayla
Dillon
Luke
Avery
Mila

May this inspire you to realize
that there is no such word as "can't."

CONTENTS

FOREWORD

At the Heart and Stroke Foundation of Canada we had to face a hard truth in the mid 1990s. At that time stroke was Canada's forgotten disease—even though it was the country's fourth leading cause of death. According to a 1996 Foundation study, almost half of all Canadians said they wouldn't know what to do if they thought they were having a stroke. And only thirty-nine per cent of us could name one of stroke's most common warning signs: a feeling of numbness, sudden weakness or tingling in the face, arm and leg. At the same time, new drugs coupled with greater medical knowledge were making it possible to reduce and even reverse stroke's devastating effects—but only if people knew what was happening to them and sought and received urgent emergency medical help.

It seemed clear to us that the Foundation needed help to spread the message on stroke and we decided to commit to a major public awareness campaign. Getting the facts out is one thing. But how could we persuade people to pay attention to those facts, and take our message to heart? The Foundation needed to put a special face to stroke—a face that would give Canadians the knowledge and the courage to recognize and react immediately when they suspected stroke. An instantly recognizable face, of a person who would be highly respected and credible in carrying a message of hope for those recovering from stroke, their families, and indeed, for all Canadians.

Who better to help the Foundation in this mission than Walter Gretzky?

When he had his life-threatening stroke on October 13, 1991, it seemed as if the whole country was waiting for news about his recovery. As his family members flew in to be at his bedside, the prognosis was grim. But Walter battled back, with the help of excellent medical care, dedicated therapists and the love and grit of his family. Not only was he leading a full life but he was constantly giving back to charities and communities. Would he help us?

We were nervous as we stood at the Gretzky doorstep in Brantford, Ontario, on a blustery December day in 1999. We were there to make the Foundation's pitch, but we also knew we were joining a long line of organizations that had sought the endorsement of the Gretzky family to help get their messages heard. What if Walter said no?

We didn't know then that the word Walter has the hardest time saying is "No."

Walter Gretzky exudes human kindness and caring. If Walter

thinks he can make a difference in just one person's life, he's there without question. He has a remarkable sense of duty to others, and often pushes aside his own needs and personal reservations whenever a gesture on his part—big or small—has a chance to evoke a feeling of hope or even a smile. After five minutes in his presence, we understood how strangers can quickly become so comfortable with him and why they often turn up on his doorstep to ask him to visit a relative who's suffered a stroke.

But he's humble. He'll chat about hockey, about coaching kids, about the big events in Wayne's career, about his pride in all his children and grandchildren. He'll tell funny stories about things that have happened to him on the road and about the way he likes to tease his wife, Phyllis. But he couldn't understand why anyone would be interested in the details of his life or think he was some kind of expert on stroke. In his eyes, he was just an ordinary hard-working down-to-earth guy from Brantford to whom some extraordinary things had happened: like coming back not once but twice from brushes with death and raising the only hockey player in the history of the game called the Great One.

When the Foundation made the case that if Walter went public with his story someone might listen to his message and get to the hospital in time, he agreed to get involved. If his words could help save even one life, it would be worth it. And once Walter was involved, being Walter, he put his whole heart into it.

That initial public service campaign became a springboard to countless other activities Walter has undertaken for the Foundation in its fight against stroke. From a "Dear Walter" newspaper column, to media tours, to fundraisers, Walter has travelled this country tirelessly to get our life-saving stroke messages heard.

Overcoming his real humility in order to publicly recount his personal journey back from stroke in this book speaks volumes to his unwavering commitment to helping others. The lasting impact from Walter's stroke was on his memory, and telling his life story meant once again having to confront what he has lost. One night driving with his publisher from the family farm back to his house in Brantford, he summed it up for her: "I just have to think of it this way. Yes, I've forgotten some of the good times, and I'll never get those memories back. But I must have forgotten a lot of bad times too, and that's a blessing!"

There are many people who must be acknowledged for helping to bring this book to life. First and foremost, the Gretzky family— Phyllis, Wayne, Kim, Keith, Glen and Brent, and Ian Kohler, Kim's husband and Walter's former rehabilitation specialist. Special thanks must go to Glen, Kim and Ian, who were instrumental in turning the dream of this book into a reality, and had the foresight to realize that Walter's story could be a source of hope and inspiration for other stroke survivors and their families.

At Random House Canada, we thank the publisher, Anne Collins, and rights and contracts vice president Jennifer Shepherd for their expert counsel at every juncture along the way. We are also grateful to Moira Farr for her ability to help Walter catch the memories of a life on paper.

At the Heart and Stroke Foundation, we acknowledge the contributions of Dr. Ken Buchholz, Sharon Edwards, Dr. Gail Eskes,

Elissa Freeman, Karen Fedun, Rick Gallop, Tim Julien, Gail Leadlay, Mary Lewis, Doug MacQuarrie, Scott Ogilvie, Sylvia Poirier, Dr. Frank Silver, Richard Sutherland and Dr. Michele Turek.

Diane Black   Frank Rubini

HEART AND STROKE FOUNDATION

One of Walter's favourite sayings is, "Every moment of every day is precious to me." For those of us at the Foundation who've come to know Walter, every day he has been our stroke crusader has been precious to us.

Whenever people meet me, they are usually very curious to know, "What's it like being Wayne Gretzky's dad?" Wayne is my oldest son, of course, a pretty good hockey player whose name may ring a bell for you. He's retired from the ice now, but he's still managing to keep himself busy. I guess he inherits that, along with his love of hockey, from his dad. It's a question I get asked all the time, and in response, I say that mostly it's been fantastic beyond my wildest dreams. It's given me the chance to travel widely, meet amazing people and do things that I never would have had the opportunity to do otherwise. I love to tell stories, and believe me, these experiences have given me some good ones! It's all been a great adventure, and I've been happy to share it with my family and friends.

Naturally, I feel enormous pride, as any father would, in my son's accomplishments. People often seem to think I had something to do with those, but I always say, when it comes to talent like that, it seems to me there's some destiny involved. I just did what I could to help it along. And really, the thing I am most proud of is the fact that apart from being a great hockey player, Wayne's a great person off the ice. As a parent, that's what you most want to be able to say about your kids, in my opinion. When I talk about feeling lucky, that's what I mean, more than anything else.

I'll be honest with you, though: sometimes all the fame and celebrity that go with being related to the guy they call the greatest hockey player who ever lived have been a challenge—for Wayne, for me and for the whole Gretzky family. It's a privilege but also a responsibility that has to be handled carefully. Living so close to the spotlight, you can be a magnet for some pretty strange things, and we've certainly seen it all: the good, the bad and the ugly. We have tried to take it all in stride and keep things in perspective. Fans of Wayne would be disappointed if we didn't. We all appreciate that if it weren't for those fans, we wouldn't enjoy the kind of life we do.

But with all the relentless focus on Wayne over the years, people tend to forget the whole picture. The fact is, I've been the proud dad of four other great kids, too: Kim, Glen, Keith and Brent, the latter two both talented hockey players in their own right. I've also been the grateful husband, for the past forty-one years, of a wonderful woman, Phyllis, and granddad to twelve (at last count) members of the new generation. Away from the limelight, we Gretzkys have a fulfilling family life that we cherish and protect.

I'd say, more than anything, we are ordinary people who have had some extraordinary things happen to us. Maybe that's why so many others feel comfortable approaching me and telling me their own stories—and I've heard them all, including some very sad ones. Whether I'm at home or on the road, I do what I can to help. Sometimes, I've noticed, all people really want is someone to listen to them and to show some caring and compassion. I'm happy to do this whenever I can, especially when I see that a person is having a rough time getting over a big hurdle in his or her life, through no fault of their own. There are many people out there, especially kids, who deserve a helping hand.

You have to understand, I have a very down-to-earth background. My parents were immigrants to this country. They had no money, they simply came and were grateful to quietly put down roots and work hard all their lives to give their children a good home and a good start in life. I'm really just a country kid at heart. If someone had told me back when I was growing up on our little cucumber farm in Canning, near Brantford, that one day I'd be travelling all over the world, meeting prime ministers and presidents, hobnobbing with all sorts of remarkable people, both famous and not so famous, I would have said, "No way!" Sometimes, I swear to you, I have to pinch myself to make sure I'm not dreaming. Wayne says the same thing. People call him the Great One, but he's remarked on more than one occasion that he's really the Grateful One.

Wayne's phenomenal success has brought on a lot of public curiosity about us, but still, I have to admit, when people suggested that I write a book telling the story of my life, the idea was a little foreign to me. So much has been written about Wayne, why would anyone be interested in a whole book about me? I'm just a guy who grew up on a farm, worked for Bell Canada for thirty-four years and raised a sport-loving family in a small Canadian town. It doesn't seem very remarkable.

But something out of the ordinary did happen to me back in 1991, which changed the course of my life dramatically. I had a brain aneurysm, or stroke, that nearly did me in. Truly, when it happened, I wasn't supposed to live through the night. I was only fifty-three years old at the time and just a few months into a retirement I had been dreaming about. Believe me, recovering from that stroke wasn't easy. It was a devastating blow to our family. None of us could have known back then what a long and painful journey it was going to be. Once I'd woken up from the surgery, my work was cut out for me. I literally had to start from square one, trying to figure out who and where I was, and how I was going to get my life back. This is a fairly common problem after a stroke. The worst part was that I lost a great deal of my memory and my capacity to retain new memories. It was not easy coming to terms with this loss, for me or my loved ones. In fact, for awhile it was downright depressing. It took a very long time for me to become independent again. I had to go through many phases of recovery, which was gradual and, at times, very frustrating. I was physically weak at first and extremely confused. The truth is, I hardly remember a thing about the first three years or so after my stroke. I know it was hard on my family. They like to say that I was "sleeping" through that period. When I don't remember something from that time, they'll say, "Dad, that happened while you were still sleeping. It happened before you woke up."

Well, as luck would have it, the stroke didn't kill me, and here I am, ten years later, healthy, happy and eternally grateful that I can tell any story at all! I try to be philosophical and accept the reality of what's happened. You have to do that if you are going to move on from that kind of setback. Difficult as it has been, with the love and support of my family and many other dedicated people in my life, I have regained my independence and have learned how to cope with difficulties I have with short-term memory, and those gaps in my long-term memory, which include most of the '80s and the majority of Wayne's career highlights.

So many memories were lost to me with the stroke! It's a strange feeling, to stare at a photograph of yourself from a decade or more ago, and say, "Gee, I guess that really happened," because there I am, but I honestly have no recollection of the event. Sometimes, people approach me in public and, not being aware of my problem, will start talking about a time we met back in the '80s. Of course, they assume I'll remember and be able to engage in their reminiscences. But most of the time, I'm sorry to say, I just don't have access to those memories; they're really gone for good. It sounds sad, but I look at it this way: it's unfortunate that there are good things I don't remember from the past, but then again, there's a lot of not-so-great things I can't remember, either. You could say that's a blessing too!

People who know me well say I'm a different guy now than I was before the stroke. I guess I'd have to agree with them. The changes are fairly obvious. For one thing, I used to hate the game of golf, and now you'd have a hard time getting me off the course! Joking aside, I am a lot more outgoing and less serious than I used to be. I wasn't all that keen on public speaking before, though I would do it when called upon; now I just love being up in front of an audience. I never envisioned my retirement unfolding this way, but I'm busier than ever with speaking engagements across the country, and I love being on the move, meeting new people, sharing my stories and hearing theirs. You cannot imagine what a blessing it is for me to be able to do this. I'm having the time of my life! After my stroke ten years ago, and for several years following, I don't think I or anyone in my family would have thought it possible that I'd be where I am today. That is what fills all of us with gratitude.

Most significantly, I'd say the greatest change of all is that I don't worry about the little things in life the way I did before. And worrying really was a big part of my life for a long, long time. All that just seems to have been swept away, which I consider to be a good thing, too. I enjoy life now, much more than I ever did before. Why not? I guess I have a sense of how short and how precious our lives really are, and I want to get the most out of mine and offer what I can to others I meet along the way.

I'm grateful, so many years after my aneurysm, to have this opportunity to look back on my life, before and after, piecing together the memories I do have—some, especially from childhood and my early life, are very vivid to me—and, with help, reconstructing all the other events of my life. You might find out some things about me here that will surprise you. I hope you will find this book entertaining and that you'll enjoy hearing my stories as much as I enjoy telling them.

———

A lot of people helped in creating this book, and I thank them: family members and friends who assisted me with their own recollections of incidents from my early life, and people who were key to my recovery, especially Ian Kohler, my rehabilitation therapist and now a member of our family, too—but I'll let him tell you how that came about in the chapters concerning my rehabilitation in hospital and at home, in which he played an essential role. In fact, I trust Ian so much, I've let him tell much of the story of what happened during the early weeks, months and years of my recovery. He was there, every step of the way, and I can't thank him enough for all the help he gave me, along with my wife, Phyllis, my daughter, Kim, and my sons, Wayne, Keith, Glen and Brent. I must extend a warm thank-you to Sandi McLean, Phyllis's sister, who was a pillar of strength and a stabilizing force for Phyllis and Kim at a critical time during my recovery. Without a moment's hesitation she would drop whatever she was doing to assist in any way possible. A special thanks to Butch Steele, Eddie Ramer and Ron Finucan, who stood by Phyllis and Kim through my days and nights in the hospital, and through the years of my rehabilitation. Other friends and neighbours who helped along the way: Charlie Henry, Warren MacGregor, Mary and Sil Rizzetto and Karen Redpath. I owe a deep debt of gratitude to Laurie Ham, who just happened to be the guardian angel who got me to the hospital in time for treatment, and Dr. Rocco de Villiers, the neurosurgeon at Hamilton General Hospital who saved my life.

I'd also like to thank the people at the Heart and Stroke Foundation of Canada, especially Frank Rubini, who was the person who recruited me to the Heart and Stroke Foundation. He persuaded me that writing this book would be a great idea, in the belief that people would read about my experience and understand more about Canada's fourth largest killer. He also felt it would be an invaluable resource for stroke survivors and their families. With his determination and optimism, Frank has been with me and my family every step of the way in making this book a reality. He has also spent many a day and night travelling the country with me on national media tours and public awareness campaigns to make Canadians aware of the signs and symptoms of stroke. I know that our work has helped to save lives across the country. Thanks also to Diane Black, who bridged the gap between HSFC and Random House Canada in producing the book. I was convinced that by telling my story of recovery from stroke, I might help someone else who could be ignoring some very significant signs or symptoms— just like I had! All of these people I've just mentioned and many others are responsible for allowing me to continue living a full and rewarding life.

"Amazing Grace" is my favourite hymn. I think after you read this book, you'll understand why. I feel like I've been given a second chance at life, and I don't want to waste a second of it. I really do enjoy every day I have on this earth now. I try not to take myself too seriously, nor do I take any of the good things I've been given for granted. Most of all, I believe you can't go wrong in life if you just try your best, whatever it is you choose to do and whatever the level of your abilities. I've always believed that and have tried to pass it on to my own kids as well as all those kids I've coached over the years. You can go a long way with that attitude, even when the deck seems stacked against you. It is a wonderful life, if you decide to make it that way. After all the hard times I and my family have been through as a result of my stroke, I can still wholeheartedly say that. Every day is full of surprises, and I genuinely look forward to every one. Ten years ago, I wouldn't have been able to say that. If what I offer, in telling my story here, is a message of hope for even one person struggling with similar difficulties, or any kind of disability at all, I will feel that the effort has been worthwhile.

chapter one

A COUNTRY BOY

Home for me when I was growing up was a little white farm-house on the banks of the Nith River, in a rural community called Canning, not too far from my current home in Brantford, Ontario. Even today, when I think of home, my mind fills with memories of that old house by the river. It would be true to say it remains at the heart of our family's story, and that we all think of it as a special place. My daughter, Kim, lives there with her young family today. She swears the ghost of my mother, Mary Gretzky, watches over the house still. Knowing my mother, I believe that.

The Gretzky farm wasn't very big, just thirty-three acres, but it was typical of the family farms in the area at the time. The house was built in 1831—in fact, it was once the town's one and only hotel—when Canning was a prosperous and growing community and everyone was hoping that the train would eventually come through. Instead, the tracks went to nearby Paris, and Canning became a quiet, rural settlement instead of a bustling town.

Like everyone else in the area, we grew our own fruit and vegetables and were self-sufficient when it came to feeding ourselves. My mother was a great cook, and I remember eating very well— good, old-country, Polish food. Her perogies—pronounced *pera-ha* in our house—were second to none (and in her honour, Wayne has put them on the menu at his restaurant in Toronto). My father, who was from Russia, made great wine. Having a glass of wine with your meal is part and parcel of growing up in a European culture. His remedy for a cold, and a good remedy it is, was to heat up some wine and drink it with tea. Add lemon and sugar, that's it. Cure your cold, absolutely!

We had chickens, ducks, cows and pigs. We sold milk from the cows, raised our own feed and had our own eggs. We also ate fish regularly from the river, mostly pike and bass. Bass were the best. I loved fishing. I'd go in the morning and wouldn't come back until late at night. I'd row up and down the river in an old boat. My mother would clean and cook the fish we brought home, and they made up the most delicious meals I can remember. Back then, you could eat as much fish as you wanted out of the river. I carried my love of fishing into adulthood and have spent many a peaceful time with buddies of mine out there casting. I don't do it as much now, but I used to go every weekend. I loved taking the kids out, nieces and nephews included, and teaching them how to fish, too.

We also occasionally hunted and trapped on our property— just small game, like rabbits or muskrat—but I didn't continue with the hunting. My brother Albert tells me he never touched a gun after an incident that happened when we were young teenagers. We were prowling the woods out back of the farm when he accidentally took a shot that narrowly missed me. I had no idea what a close call it was until he told me himself. I was very thankful, as I'm sure the rabbit who got away that day was, too.

We had an old-fashioned, rural life. Helping us out on the farm was a big old plowhorse named Bob. We were all very fond of that horse, and it was a sad day when he died after choking on a stalk of corn. Everybody will tell you how good that horse was. So gentle. He would stand there on the front lawn, and my little sister, Ellen, would walk between his legs. My mother would tell the rest of us not to run or we'd scare the horse and he'd step on our baby sister. But Bob never hurt Ellen or anyone else.

On a regular day, we had our chores to do before we went to school. There were cows to milk, and the hay had to be put down for them. We had to make sure all the animals were fed. During harvest time, most of the local kids would leave school to work in the fields. On our farm, we'd pick cucumbers from dawn till dusk. The whole family pitched in, and you never questioned that the work had to be done. When you live on a farm and the fields are full of vegetables in need of picking, you just have to do it or the crop rots—and my parents would never have allowed that kind of waste. Then we would take Bob all the way from Canning to Paris, hitched up to a buggy filled with cucumbers. We'd transport bags and bags of them down to the processing plant. That was our way of life. I didn't know it was work until I got to high school and met kids who didn't live on farms.

That was only fifty years ago, but when I tell my kids and grandkids what life was like back then, I know they have trouble imagining it. It was another world. No TV, no computer games, no Pokémon, no pizza delivered to the door, no designer T-shirts or running shoes. Sometimes it's hard for me to believe how different it was back then, too! We didn't have much of anything in the way of material possessions, just the basics.

Like many of the men in the area, my father worked for years at Penman's, the textile factory in nearby Paris, and his wages never reached fifty dollars a week. If we needed something, he'd work overtime. As my sister Jennie likes to say, our mother could take a dollar and squeeze it until it made two. She had no choice. It was a matter of survival. I remember bringing little peeping chicks in from the barn to the kitchen to keep them warm, because somehow they had hatched in the middle of winter—it's not supposed to happen, but it does. We kept these chicks in the kitchen, so they wouldn't freeze to death in the barn. We didn't want to lose them. That's how it was. It was that simple. Nobody thought anything of it.

By today's standards, it might seem that we were poor, but we didn't feel poor. Everyone in the community lived the same way. We had what we needed in the way of food, clothing and shelter, and we weren't aware of any other way of living. As new immigrants to Canada, my parents were just happy to have a small plot of land to call their own and a safe place where they could raise their children in peace.

My father, Tony Gretzky, had gone to Chicago from Russia before he came to Canada. His family had been landowners in the old country, supporters of the czar. When anyone asked my father if he was Russian, he'd say, "Nyet. Belarus," meaning, White Russian, the upper class. In the early years of the twentieth century, when the Russian Revolution was brewing, many White Russians living in the Ukraine saw the writing on the wall, and my grandfather was among those who decided his family should get out before it became dangerous. That was a wise move! My father ended up in the United States. When the First World War broke out and he was going to join the U.S. Army, someone said to him, "You should join the Canadian army, they treat you better." So that's what he did. He served overseas and returned to Canada afterwards. He was extremely proud of having fought for this country and was a rank-and-file member of the Paris Legion. Right into his old age, when he was very frail, he insisted on putting on his uniform and attending Remembrance Day ceremonies every year. "I have to," he'd say, "I *have* to." I don't think he missed a single one while he could still walk. He strongly believed it was his duty to honour and never forget his fallen comrades. We're very proud of Tony Gretzky ourselves. Photographs of him from his war years are prominently displayed on our walls, and we've kept his war medals.

My dad—we called him Tato—was a very calm man, gracious, the kind of person who never met a stranger. And very proud, especially when it came to his house. He felt he was as good as anybody. You could talk to him about anything. I'd say my mother was the practical one, while my father was more of a thinker and dreamer. If it weren't for my mother, I don't know that the farm would have run quite as efficiently as it did. My father did a lot of work, but she really ran the place.

Mary, my mother, came to Canada from Poland in 1928, and that's when my parents met in Toronto. They moved to the farm in Canning in 1931. They spoke Ukrainian at home, and that was my first language. Obviously, it's imprinted very deeply in me, because right after I had my stroke, that's what I was speaking when I first regained consciousness. According to my brother Albert, who was one of the few people who could understand what the heck I was saying, it was as though, in my mind, I was transported back to my early years on the farm. Apparently I kept asking whether the chickens had been fed. (You can take the boy out of the country . . .)

There were seven children in our family. I was number five, after my half-sister, Olga (who was the child of my father's first marriage and came over from Russia with him, without her mother), Edward, Sophie and Jennie. Albert came after me and then the youngest, Ellen, who was born with Down's syndrome. Al tells me I was my mother's favourite. In fact, he recalls feeling jealous of me when we were kids!

ALBERT GRETZKY: He was Mama's pet. I don't know whether Mother knew something we didn't back then. For her, when he was still a baby, he could walk on water. Oh yeah, absolutely.

I mean that in a nice way, now. I didn't think so at the time. But we've overcome that. When we grew up to be adults we understood, you know, a parent's a parent, and all parents have favourites.

Mother made great pies, just incredible. Apple, pear, peach, you name it. An abundance. But if there was raisin pie and that's all there was left, for my brother, who didn't like raisin pie, well, she would make one special, so he didn't have to eat it. The rest of us had to eat it, but he got peach or cherry, whatever.

I do admit that my mother treated me very well, that we had a great bond. I've lost a lot of memories as a result of my stroke, but one from childhood that remains completely vivid is walking by my mother's side—I must have been five or six—holding her hand, as she took me to the one-room schoolhouse a mile up the road for the first day of school. I remember her telling me very firmly and repeatedly not to be scared. And walking beside her like that, I wasn't.

I have the utmost admiration and respect for what my mother went through to raise her family, all the hard work she did every day of her life. I never asked her if this story is true, but my understanding is that she gave birth to at least one of her children in the house and then was back in the field working, the same day. She was a strong woman who did what she had to to get by and didn't complain about her lot in life. She was a devout Roman Catholic and her moral code ruled in our little farmhouse on the river. She was the disciplinarian in the family, very strict with us and very clear about the standards of behaviour we had to meet. To this day, I can never walk through a door before a lady, because I would get a cuff across the head from my mother if I ever showed such disrespect. To her, it was essential that we prove ourselves to be upstanding and equal members of the community. Like so many immigrants, she must have struggled with the sense of being an outsider when she arrived in Canada. In the early years, she couldn't speak English, though she eventually learned it from all of us and got to the point where she could speak it, read the paper and watch TV, understanding everything. I remember when Mama turned eighty-four. She had a quick wit, and when a reporter asked her, "Well Mrs. Gretzky, how does it feel to be eighty-four?" she said, "I don't know, I've never been eighty-four before." I thought that was just a fantastic answer. She'd come a long way, being able to deliver a response like that. In the beginning, when my father was at work and us kids were at school, she'd hide if someone came knocking at the door, because she couldn't speak English. I think she felt intimidated by our English-speaking Canadian neighbours, although many were immigrants just like us. There was a mix of ethnic groups: Dutch, German, Hungarian, Slovakian, Ukrainian, everything.

As far as my mother was concerned, her kids were just as good as anyone else and we deserved every opportunity to make something of ourselves. In that way, she really encouraged us, as did my dad, to work hard and do our best in whatever pursuits we chose. This huge commitment she had to her family, her forceful personality and her strong belief system had an impact on all of us, I think, and our own kids, too. That's why it doesn't surprise me when my daughter, Kim, who went to live in the house with my mother and Ellen for several years before my mother died in 1988, tells me she's sure her grandmother's ghost is still there.

My mother used to sit in a rocking chair in the corner of the kitchen, reading the newspaper—Kim swears that when she walks in there sometimes, she can hear paper rattling. One time, Kim put a kettle on the stove and turned on the burner, then left the kitchen for a couple of minutes. When she got back, the burner had been turned off. There was no one else in the house, and Kim is not old enough to be forgetful like me. When she told me this, I said, "You know, your grandmother just hated it when anyone would put the stove on and leave the room."

Finally, Kim has witnessed some very strange behaviour in one of her dogs. My mother couldn't stand to see dogs in the house, but Kim allows hers inside. Once, when her dog went in what had been my mother's bedroom, he seemed agitated and avoided the side of the bed she used to sleep on, as though someone was still there! People have asked Kim whether she feels scared, and she says, "Why would I be scared? It's Grandma. She's just looking after us, the way she always did."

I learned to be protective of my sister Ellen from an early age. All of my siblings did. It's an old saying, and unfortunately true: kids can be cruel. We accepted Ellen as she was, but people's attitudes towards those with mental and physical disabilities were so different back then. There was a lot of misunderstanding, a sense of shame that was attached to a family with a child like Ellen, though I don't remember ever feeling that. Families with Down's syndrome children had to either take care of them as best they could, or sign them away to an institution forever, where they'd be looked after by strangers. My mother certainly wasn't going to allow that to happen. It simply wouldn't have entered her mind. But she never really understood or accepted that Ellen was the way she was from before birth, either. Ellen fell and hit her head as a baby, and my mother was convinced that that fall caused her to be the way she was.

We did the best we could. I remember thinking it would be a good idea for Ellen to attend the one-room schoolhouse along with the rest of us. Mrs. Dafoe, the teacher, was a wonderful, smiling, red-headed woman, very kind, whose husband started one of the first tobacco farms in the area. She was an absolute angel. I persuaded her to let Ellen come, and for a few years, she did. I'd usually walk Ellen to school, and Albert would walk her home. I did have to stand up for her sometimes and defend her against the kids' teasing. I would always do that.

I try to imagine how difficult this was: to let Ellen go out into the world, in public, for everybody to see, this child who wasn't "right." That was really big. You have to remember, we're talking about a community of people from the "old country," with old-country ways and beliefs that we would find strange today.

I'm sure it was hard for Mrs. Dafoe, too, who probably had thirty other students to teach in that one room, at every elementary grade level. But she let Ellen run around and amuse herself while she was there. Unfortunately, when Mrs. Dafoe left, the new teacher wasn't so fond of the idea, and so Ellen stopped going to school and spent her days back at the farm with my mother.

Ellen has the mental capacity of a four-year-old and needs help with everything, from feeding herself to getting dressed to combing her hair. She has to be supervised at all times, and we had some pretty scary close calls when she wasn't. I'll never forget the time when she got hold of an old inner tube and managed to push herself out into the river. The rest of us used to swim there all the time, bobbing around on inner tubes, no problem, but my mother had gathered them up and put them away in a shed, because she knew they could be a hazard for Ellen. Somehow, when she was around fourteen years old, Ellen got her hands on an old tire, which to her looked a lot like the inner tubes we all used. She went down to the river and got herself in, and the tire started filling with water, and began to sink. She was just a tiny little thing and when my mother spotted her, her head was just at the surface of the water. My mum managed to grab her and get her back to shore, but that was a big fright, and we knew we had to watch her all the more closely after that.

My mother was devoted to Ellen's care and, in her old age, became afraid of what might happen to her when she passed away. "I hope she dies the second after I do," she would say, scared that Ellen would end up neglected or mistreated. She didn't have to worry, though, because we all wanted to make sure Ellen was well looked after. Today, she lives with Phyllis and me and sometimes goes down to stay for periods of time with Jennie, who moved to North Carolina with her American husband, Paul Hopper, many years ago. Jenny met Paul when he came up to Canning to help the Dafoes get their tobacco farm going back in the early '50s. They have three grown kids of their own now, and our families have been close, despite the geographical distance between us. I was always fond of Jennie, who is just a few years older than me. When she left school and took a job in Paris, I remember my mother wasn't too pleased. She thought Jennie should continue her education. I also remember that whenever Jennie got paid, she'd give me a little bit of spending money.

Just one more thing about Ellen: I've always said she has a sixth sense about people. I watch how she is with anyone who comes to the door, and her reaction is a bit of a gauge for me of what a person is like. If Ellen is comfortable around someone, if she isn't afraid and gives them a hug, I feel I can trust that person. But if she shies away or seems wary of them in any way, I take note of that. It's nature's protection of her, and for all that she's mentally disabled, she's got pretty good "people radar."

Our family has been blessed with many individuals of exceptional talent, but I think Ellen has taught us compassion and the ability to accept people as they are. We all firmly believe that everyone has something special to contribute, including those with mental and physical challenges. Many people know that Wayne developed a special relationship with a boy who has Down's syndrome, Joey Moss, when he was playing with the Oilers in Edmonton. Wayne's also done a lot to raise money over the years, through his tennis and golf tournaments, to help visually challenged kids. As a family, we are all proud to be associated with the Canadian National Institute for the Blind (CNIB) and to help in any way we can. I know Wayne and all my kids got a good part of their caring attitude and sense of responsibility toward more vulnerable people from being around Ellen.

Back in the old days, when I was growing up, we had to look after ourselves, and I think we did a pretty good job. Like I said, we were typical of the families in the area. My parents had some good friends in the community, people like the Kischaks, who had eight children, next door to us. Mrs. Kischak, a widow now in her eighties, still lives there on her own, and I like to drop in to visit with her now and then. Her son Steve, who unfortunately passed away not too long ago, was a good buddy of mine. I'll never forget, one of our favourite things to do together was run. I don't mean on a track (that came later), I mean all along the concession roads around our homes. We'd make a game of it, just loping along at full tilt for as long we could. We'd literally run for miles and miles, just a couple of farm boys with nothing better to do than burn off energy. I remember we'd land back at our place and collapse, laughing and laughing. It wasn't a bad way to amuse yourself, when you think of it. Cost nothing, too.

The river was a big part of our lives. There were rapids, a swimming hole not far down from us and a great big weeping willow tree with a rope attached to it, which the kids used to swing out on and plunge into the river. I nearly drowned myself one time. I can remember hanging there on the rope when I was little, the water eight or nine feet deep below me, and I was hollering and hollering. A guy who was coming to see my older brother, Ed, was standing on the bridge. Next thing I knew, I was on the bank. I must have finally fallen in. From the bridge, that fellow ran all the way down to the swimming hole, which is about a hundred yards away, and pulled me out. I guess kids were always getting into trouble around there. On summer days, whole families and groups of people would have picnics, fish and just relax on the banks. That was a really big deal, seeing everybody there from all the little communities around us.

An even bigger deal would be our occasional car trips to Toronto, to visit with friends of my parents, and with Olga, who had married and moved there with her husband and kids. Today, that trip takes roughly an hour, but back then, it was more like four, one way. Tato was a slow and cautious driver (I've been accused of being the same myself). I remember he'd always drive with the headlights on, and when I asked him why, he said this was to alert people that we were coming from a long way away!

I remember some of the parties the adults would have. Lots of food, laughter and music—most of it Eastern European. My dad had an old Russian mandolin he'd play while he sang, and he was an amazing dancer, too. When he got going, in that Cossack style, his legs would fly so fast, honestly, it looked like he was floating above the ground!

We all got involved in music one way or another at school. In fact, Albert and I were not a bad little duo for awhile there, singing in competitions like the Kiwanis Festival. I don't know where the certificates are now, but I know that when we were about eight or ten (Al's two years younger than me), we were judged the best duo for our age group in the county. In fact, we ended up in a specially chosen choir of area kids who sang for the king and queen (now the Queen Mother) when they came to visit Canada in the late '40s. The music teacher, Mr. Ferguson, who came around to all the schools once a month, picked us and a few others to go, and we stood on the platform at the railway station in Woodstock, Ontario, and sang our little hearts out as the royal train passed through. I guess Albert and I never made it to the big time with our act, and it's too late now, but I've always enjoyed singing and still do.

Music was fun, but my biggest thrill was definitely sports. I don't know where the interest and ability comes from in our family, to tell you the truth. My parents weren't involved in athletics. I was never a big guy, but I was agile. My brother Al claims that I got out of a few brushes with the leather strap because I could outrun anyone who came at me with one. I guess all those hell-bent runs with Steve Kischak must have paid off.

> ALBERT: Walter was an athlete right from public school. Ran like a deer. Just phenomenal . . . with him, it was speed to burn.

By the time I was in my teens, I was a member of the track and field team at Paris High School. I set a few records in running, long jump and pole vault, and I think some of those records stood for quite awhile too, if I'm not mistaken. I used to make my own poles from trees on our property. I'd just walk into the bush, pick a long, tall tree I thought looked particularly good for the purpose and chop it down. Sounds primitive, but it worked.

Back then, I was athletic, but also a pretty serious student, keen to get good grades and be involved with as many school activities as possible. There were about four hundred students at my high school, from all around the Paris area, and I think most of us had pretty positive attitudes about doing our best and respecting our teachers. We worked hard, enjoyed what we were doing. We didn't have anything called a late bus. If you wanted to be involved in after-school activities, you just had to find your way home somehow. Most kids did live way out in the country, but we managed. Someone on the team might have a motorcycle and agree to drop you off. Someone else would borrow the family car, or a parent might pick you up. I remember when I missed the bus, I'd walk from the high school down to Penman's and get a ride with my dad. And sometimes we'd arrange it so he could pick me up. One day, my dad was going to pick me up at the school around 5:15. I decided to wait for him in the downstairs washroom, where there was a bench I could lie down on. I must have been very tired, because I fell fast asleep. When my dad arrived and I wasn't outside waiting for him, he went into the school to look for me. He and the janitor finally found me all curled up and out cold on the bench.

The track team was known as the Boys' Athletic Association, and we were a winning team, provincially. Apart from the track team, if you can believe it, I served on the yearbook committee one year. I actually typed out the entire thing, using the famous one-finger technique. My yearbook nickname was "Manager Gretzky," and my friends had this to say about me: "Walter is a studious boy, getting extra marks from JC." (I am sure these were the initials of a teacher, not of the good Lord himself.) It's true I was manager of the basketball team, even though I didn't know anything about basketball. Our gym teacher, Gerry Barnhill, said that was okay, I could still do the job. I think I had a spare fifteen minutes in my schedule, so I had to fill it up. Mainly, I used to post the scores from the game on the bulletin board.

ALBERT: Walter's kind of like Wayne, you know, he had everything. He was smart, he had talent, all the girls were after him because he had all that, and he was a track star. You'd watch, and he'd win the 100 yard dash or the steeplechase, the high jump, pole vault. On and on. Then there was hockey. Was he good? You bet . . .

While I loved track and excelled at it, I have to admit that my greatest love was hockey. I grew up playing it on the river behind the house. That was the number one sport for us back then. Really, from a pretty early age, I couldn't get enough of it. Couldn't wait for the river to freeze over so I could get out on that ice. Coming from a little place like Canning, you really had to teach yourself how to do things and just hope you had some natural talent. Of course, in the beginning, the games were casual, just a bunch of local boys playing around. Al would be goaltender, I'd be forward line. But then when I was about fourteen, I got onto a local team and started playing in arenas around Canning and Paris. Some of them were pretty terrible by today's standards. The Drumbo arena—a horrific place! There's never been anything like it, before or since. So cold you might as well have been outside, and it seemed to be built for tiny people—the taller players could hit their heads on the beams! But that's all you had in those days, and if you wanted to play hockey, you put up with it.

When I was in my later teens, I played Junior B with the Woodstock Warriors. I wasn't a big guy, maybe five-foot-nine, 140 pounds tops. I can remember playing with my friend Warren MacGregor in the nearby town of Ayr. We were on the same line, and there was a guy on the other team who was twice the size of me. He was the centreman, and every time I came up, he'd give me a jab with his stick or elbow. Warren said to me, "I'll try to talk to that guy." He went over, and the guy hauled off and hit Warren before he got a chance to say anything. Warren came staggering back, and I asked, "What did he say?" Warren said, "He wants to talk to you." I thought that was kind of funny.

Warren used to tease me, saying, "I spend all the time in the corner, and you get all the glory." You know, he'd get the broken nose, I'd get the goal.

WARREN MacGREGOR: In track and field, Wally was better than a lot of us were, but his forte was hockey. He was a good player. I think it's inborn, the talent. Some people are just like that, more intense than others. But he was just too tiny, you know. You have to have the desire to develop your talent. He had more than his share of desire. He would play till he was just exhausted. That's where Wayne gets it from, his dad . . . Of course, we never envisioned any of this stuff was going to happen back in those days. Nobody had any idea . . .

We had fun back then, but Warren's right: I was pretty intense about it, too. I would have liked to play in the NHL, and there were a few people around who thought I might have a chance. I don't recall the man's name, but there was a local car salesman who figured that this kid was on his way to the big leagues, and he gave me a '49 Ford to drive. Actually, it wasn't a matter of giving it to me, but the purchase agreement on it was something like a dollar down, a dollar a week. I was seventeen, and a car was a pretty coveted thing. My brother Al borrowed it once, and only recently confessed he was responsible for scratching it. I let him take it out to impress his girlfriend, Marilyn—who later became (and still is) his wife—and he decided to give her a driving lesson. They were on a gravel road, a country road, and she put that car in the ditch. I didn't spot the scratch until two days later. I asked about the mark on the side of the car: "Where the hell did it come from?" Nobody confessed. Forty-five years later, Albert finally told me, and I've forgiven him. And Marilyn.

That car would soon be replaced by my beloved old Blue Goose anyway, but I'll tell that story later.

I kept my NHL dreams alive throughout my teens, and eventually I did go up to Toronto and try out for the Marlies, in the Junior A league. That must have been in '54 or '55. But I was out of luck. A couple of weeks before the trials, I got chicken pox. I was really sick, lost a lot of weight, and, as Warren said, I wasn't big to begin with. That ended up being the problem. I scored as many goals as the others did in the exhibition game, but I just wasn't big enough. I went back to playing with Woodstock.

Albert says I was good at everything, but I really had to work at school to do well. I wasn't sure what I wanted to do with my life besides sports. When I first graduated from high school, I continued to live at the farm through the summer and into the fall, picking tobacco in the neighbours' fields, which was really back-breaking work. When that was all done for the season, I was out of a job and didn't really have any idea of what I was going to do. Walking down the street in Paris one day, it must have been late September or October, I ran into Warren. When he heard I was looking for work, he told me I should apply at Bell Canada in Brantford, where he was working on the construction crew. That's exactly what I did. It was the beginning of a thirty-four-year career with Bell, for both Warren and me, and, as a matter of fact, the two of us maintained our friendship and retired on exactly the same day, back in 1991.

Once again, I have to comment on how different life was back then. I remember that around the time I started working for Bell, I was about eighteen and my mother asked me, "Walter, do you smoke?" At the time, I didn't, and so I said no. It sounds hard to believe, in light of what we know about how harmful and addictive smoking is, but she said to me, "All men smoke, you should take it up." So I did! And I was a chain-smoker right up until I had the stroke in 1991. That, and only that, was what stopped me. The surgeon who operated on me told my family that the smoking was definitely a factor in what had happened to me. And though I never did smoke again, I can tell you that I wanted to for a long time. Even during the time after the stroke that I hardly remember, the habit was so ingrained that I used to pat my pockets looking for my pack of smokes, and I'd ask for a cigarette from others whenever I had the chance. That went on for quite some time.

But way back when, my tobacco habit just made me one of the crowd, a grown-up and, according to my mother, a real man! Because I was a hyper kind of person anyway, it was easy enough for me to become a heavy smoker, just to use up some of that nervous energy, though of course it didn't really help. It was, in fact, terribly unhealthy.

It amazes me when Albert says I was popular with the girls—I really can't remember that!

I do remember meeting one particular girl, named Phyllis, at a wiener roast on the farm, which was attended by a bunch of kids from the area. She was fifteen at the time and I was eighteen. What can I say? I took one look and knew she was the one for me. I guess she felt the same way, because eventually she said yes. We got married three years after that—and forty-one years later, we're still together.

Phyllis was a very attractive, strong-willed and popular girl. Her little sister Sandi tells me now that Phyllis used to sneak out of the house after the lights were out. I swear, it was never because of me. Actually, she came to the wiener roast where we met with another boy, but I didn't let that stop me.

Phyllis was born and raised in Paris. She comes from good British stock, from down in Queenston Heights near Niagara Falls, and is a descendant of General Brock. At first her father wasn't too happy to find out she was planning to marry someone who didn't share their heritage. I'd be lying if I said this didn't cause us some friction in the beginning, but eventually we sorted it out and I was fully accepted into the family. Again, those were such different times.

Really, we were just typical small-town kids in the '50s: pretty certain we'd find a match in our crowd, get married and start having kids without delay. In the meantime, we amused ourselves one way or another, often driving places and hanging around in a group. Drive-in movies were all the rage then, and we'd go to lots of them in my car. And then there was the Calico Kitchen, the biggest teen hangout for miles around. It was one of those places where you ordered your food through a speaker and ate it in your car. The parking lot was gigantic. It's where you went on a Saturday night to show off your car and your girl. It was definitely the place to be seen, and it had the world's greatest foot-long hot dogs.

Other than hanging around the Calico Kitchen, Phyllis would come to see me play hockey during the season. She'd never boast, but she was a good athlete herself. Her sport was softball, and I would go along to see her games. She was just finishing high school, and I was working whatever farm jobs I could get and putting a lot of mileage on the car while travelling to games in and around Woodstock with the Junior B team.

Ours was a small wedding at the Anglican church in Paris in 1960, and we had a party afterwards at the farm. That's how people did things back then. It was pretty modest. We didn't rent a hall or anything like that; my mother and her friends just made a nice spread of food, everybody came and had a good time, and that was it.

After we got married, we moved to Brantford and lived for a time in a rented apartment. Now, we were a young married couple: I was twenty-one and Phyllis was just eighteen. Brantford was quite a change, in lifestyle and scenery, from the farm. When I started looking for a house for us, people laughed at me and said I wasn't looking so much at the house as at the backyard, to see if it was big enough and flat enough for a skating rink. I guess those same people now think I had some foresight. But I admit it, that is how much I loved hockey. And if I was going to be living away from the river, a flooded yard out back was going to have to do. So that is what I was hoping to find: a house I could afford on my starting-out salary at Bell, with a flat yard ripe for flooding in winter. And that's exactly what I found. A good thing, too. By the time Phyllis and I moved into our home on Varadi Avenue, where we still live today, I was a chain-smoking twenty-two-year-old family man, already wondering how to make ends meet and getting a head start on my reputation as a worrywart. I still played hockey in my spare time with Warren and some of the guys from Bell on a team called the Princeton Panthers in the rural league, but I had no more dreams of my own for the NHL.

I was also the proud new father of a little baby boy named Wayne Douglas Gretzky, who, I soon figured out, liked how the world looked with a stick in his hands and a pair of skates on his feet as much as his old man did. I decided to teach him everything I knew about hockey, the sport that was already a big part of my life, and as it turned out, was always going to be.

Yes, that backyard rink turned out to be a pretty good idea after all.

chapter two

SMALL-TOWN DAD

I would never deny that I've been extremely fortunate over the years, but I have to tell you that my life as a husband and father didn't exactly get off to the luckiest start. I have no doubt that Phyllis would agree with me on this one. It was 1961. Wayne wasn't even a year old. Just a few days before we were moving from our apartment into our new house (the one with the nice, flat backyard), I had a terrible accident on the job. As much as my aneurysm changed me and made me appreciate life more, I'd say that the accident in my early twenties was the first time I was given a second chance at life.

Starting out at Bell, I was a lineman. That particular day, we were guiding a big underground cable into a manhole with a wooden frame. It was a makeshift arrangement of heavy wooden cross-arms, about eight feet long and four inches in diameter, which we could weave the cable through. We were pulling on the frame, and somehow the cable tightened and the frame got flung up from the manhole with great force. It hit the back of my head, cracked my safety helmet, fractured my skull and cut open my scalp, severing all the nerves on one side of my head. You can imagine how Phyllis felt getting that telephone call. It was touch-and-go for quite awhile. In the early days, while I was in a coma, and before I showed any signs of recovery, she was advised by the people at the hospital to call in a priest.

But in the end, thankfully, I did recover with most of my senses and faculties intact, though it took a long time, probably a couple of years. The blow from the accident left me totally deaf in my right ear. My inner ear is damaged, and that's why I stagger sometimes—I lose my balance. I hear a "shhshshshsshsh" in my ear twenty-four hours a day; it's like the sound you hear from a seashell. It can be annoying, but I just ask people to stand or sit on my good side if they're talking to me, and I guess by now I'm used to it.

I went back to work after about a year and a half, but I got transferred to a different department. I became an installer, then a repairman. Over the next three decades, I worked for the business communication services group, on teleprinters, fire alarms and special circuits, all around the Brantford area. In those early years, especially when we had to get by on the disability payments I got while I was off work, it was pretty tough sometimes to make ends meet. You had to be resourceful to get by, but both Phyllis and I came from big families, where you learned how to do that. You made do, and you didn't have a lot of extravagant needs. I've always been careful about spending money, hating to see anything go to waste. I've been teased about that a lot, but it's a habit you develop when you haven't got much to spend. It's true I once vetoed new curtains for the living room in favour of skates for the boys. Skates or drapes—could there really be a contest? A sheet over the window would do the job just as well, in my opinion.

And yes, I drove the same model Chevrolet station wagon for years, and I named each one the Blue Goose. I didn't see anything wrong with driving those cars till they had 200,000 miles on them, though I admit there was some grumbling from the back seat on the way to and from hockey practices and whatever other activities the kids got into. I remember one time when the back window wouldn't go all the way up and snow was blowing in on the seat. But the old Blue Goose was a reliable car for a family of seven, and, to be honest with you, I felt more comfortable driving that than I would have a shiny new Cadillac.

Back then, I had no idea I'd ever get a chance to drive a Cadillac. It did happen, though. I was still working at Bell, when I came home one day to find my car was gone. Another car I didn't recognize was sitting there in the driveway. I said to Phyllis, "Where the devil is my car?" She said, "Your car's in the drive-way." I said, "Phyllis, where is my damn car? I want *my* car!" She said, "You've got a new one out there." Well, sure enough, Wayne had bought us a blue Cadillac for our twenty-fifth wedding anniversary. I said, "No damn way I'm going to drive to work in a Cadillac." I was an installer! Do you know how embarrassing it was to be seen driving a Cadillac to work? The guys really levelled stares at me over that.

When our kids were little, there was nothing out of the ordinary about our family. After Wayne was born in 1961 came Kim in 1963, Keith in 1967, Glen in 1969 and finally Brent in 1972. We were elated with each new arrival, but I must admit, I got pretty blasé about the whole maternity process by the time baby number five came along—a little too blasé, I think, in Phyllis's opinion. You see, just before Brent was born, Wayne had a big minor hockey championship across the border. I wanted to go and see the game, but Phyllis didn't like the idea of me being away when her due date was so close (understandably, as I appreciate now). I said, "You're going to be all right, the baby's not due for another couple of days." So, off I went with Wayne to the game.

When we got home, there was no Phyllis. She was up in the hospital, having given birth to our fifth child in my absence. Phyllis remembers that when I walked into her room in the maternity ward, the first thing I said to her was, "We won, we won!" She looked at me like I was crazy and said, "It's a boy, Walter." I guess I have to admit that sometimes I took my devotion as a hockey dad a little too far! But of course, I welcomed my brand new son with open arms; another budding hockey player, after all.

Maybe our family was a little bigger and busier than most, but we were living a pretty typical small-town life, like all the other families around us, with dads who had regular jobs and moms who mostly did not work outside the home. Brantford was a good place to raise children. We had great neighbours, like Mary and Sil Rizzetto, whose kids grew up with ours, and who remain our friends all these years later—even though our boys put their share of pucks and balls through the Rizzettos' basement windows. Mary says you could tell the changing of the seasons by the sports equipment coming in and out of our house. Hockey might have been our favourite sport, but I encouraged my kids to get involved in other activities during the summer months. These days, it's more common for people to get their kids out training on the ice all year long, but I always thought it was better to mix it up and give them a break. For one thing, it meant that when hockey season got going in the fall, the kids were really excited about it and motivated to train, because they'd had some time away from the rink, playing other sports. And it also meant that they weren't sick of the sport by age thirteen from having played nothing but hockey every day.

In those early years of raising our families, it wasn't unusual for Sil and me to borrow some money from each other back and forth, to tide us over till our paydays. We didn't think anything of it. These are the kind of folks we came to know and trust over the years, who celebrated our kids' successes—and I don't mean just Wayne's—along with us, as we did theirs. They were always there to help out when life took more challenging turns. I don't think you can overestimate the value of people like that in your life. Just be thankful they're around and realize they're priceless. They are a part of the memories I treasure.

Times could be tough, money was scarce, the house was small, just a standard-issue wartime bungalow, and family life was hectic.

We had to put food on the table, and there was lots of hockey gear to buy—we always made sure that, if nothing else, the kids got new skates that fit them properly.

I was known as a worrier. Ask people who knew me back then to strike a typical Wally Gretzky pose, and they'll put one hand on their forehead, the other on their stomach and pace around like Groucho Marx (emphasis on the Grouch)—and don't forget the cigarette constantly burning between my fingers. I admit I didn't always eat properly, either. With my job, helping my parents at the farm and delivering all those kids to their various practices and games at any given time, not to mention my own occasional games of pick-up hockey, I can tell you that it was sometimes hard to find the time to eat. I'd just forget. There was so much to fit in.

A snapshot of the Gretzky family during the '60s and '70s, if you could get us to stand still long enough to pose, would show you a growing young family that loved sports and always had some kind of activity on the go, be it hockey, baseball, lacrosse or track and field. Sometimes, the kids' hockey games would go one after another down at the arena, in order from Peewee to Bantam, so we'd be able to watch Glen, then Keith and then Wayne in one place. Other times, we would travel around to different places watching one or the other of them play. Phyllis and I would often divide that up. I think we decided pretty early on that our kids would get equal time with us as much as possible. She'd take them to early-morning practices, since I was such a night owl and didn't like to get up, and had to go to work, anyway. And I'd go to their games.

WAYNE GRETZKY: Watching his sons play hockey was my dad's greatest thrill in life. When I see how many activities he's involved in now, I have to laugh and shake my head, because back then, you'd have to have a forklift to get him away from home, even for a day, if it was for something other than one of his kids' games. He just never took a break. His forte was how hard he worked, and how he instilled that work ethic in us. Hockey tournaments were the vacations.

We loved to do it all, but it took up a lot of time and I realize now that accommodating all the family and work responsibilities put me under a lot of stress. I'm high-strung anyway. With my habit of staying up late at night, skipping meals and chain-smoking, I guess it's no wonder that I suffered severe headaches, and ulcers too. Some nights, the pain in my head behind my right eye was so bad, I couldn't lie down in bed. I'd just sit in a reclining chair all night, dozing and trying to battle the pain, which could at times make me literally feel sick to my stomach.

When I think about some of those terrible headaches, and knowing that the doctors who operated on me after my stroke found scar tissue in the frontal lobes, I feel there must have been swelling and even bleeding in the vessels in those days. Looking back, I know I didn't have the healthiest lifestyle on the planet, and I certainly would not recommend it to anyone today! It was just go, go, go, all the time, without much thought of the effect all that stress was having on my physical state. It didn't occur to me to check with a doctor about the headaches, and I see now that that was a mistake. It's a sure sign that something could be wrong, and today, anyone with some knowledge of stroke risk would tell you to have it checked out!

No one can say for sure, but if I'd changed some of my habits back then, it's possible I could have avoided the aneurysm. I don't dwell on the past now, but I have to agree with something that Wayne said, and it's kind of funny: having that aneurysm probably added years to my life. It forced me to stop smoking, eat properly, look after myself more and stop worrying so much. The fact is, I'm healthier today, all things considered, than I was back then!

Life might have been overly stretched in those days, but I think our kids have lots of happy memories of that time, as I do. In the early years, Phyllis's sister Sandi and her husband, Marvin, used to spend almost every weekend at our place, and we enjoyed their company. (Kim remains particularly close to her Aunt Sandi.) We also saw my brother Albert and his family, and kept in touch with my sister Jennie, even though she and her family lived in North Carolina. On holidays, we'd sometimes drive down there (and you can imagine what it was like with the Blue Goose loaded with five kids on a fourteen-hour journey—no wonder I had headaches), or Jennie and her husband, Paul, and their three kids, Kenny, Donna and Danny, would come here. Those were good times. The kids had the run of a big country property with their cousins in the south, and, of course, up here there was the old place in Canning, where they could swim and run around outside all day. I really enjoyed those times myself, taking the kids fishing, showing them how to drive a tractor. My nieces and nephews took to calling me

"Big Wally," and I still get that to this day. I know they had a lot of fun playing with my kids.

Kenny, who is just a couple of years older than Wayne, grew up to be a fighter pilot with the U.S. Marine Corps; we were so proud of him when he became a member of the famous Blue Angels flying squad. When he served in the Gulf War back in 1990, Wayne was so concerned about him, he stuck an American flag logo and Kenny's initials on his L.A. Kings hockey helmet and decided to keep them there until his cousin got home. We all prayed he'd come back safely, and thankfully, he did. He lives in Dallas now, and he and Wayne are still close. We've been to visit Kenny a few times. I know Wayne also remains very fond of his Aunt Jennie and sees her home in North Carolina as a place he can go and be himself with his closest relatives, away from all the celebrity limelight, which can be difficult at times. I'm glad he has that, and that all the kids have that place and those people in their memories and in their hearts. This is what really matters in life.

People tell me I could be pretty serious and intense before my stroke, much quieter than I am now. My kids say I expected a lot of them, and that is true; ours was definitely a "wait until your father gets home" kind of household. I didn't hesitate to let them know when their behaviour or attitude did not measure up. "You didn't want to disappoint Dad," is how my daughter, Kim, puts it, though she says in hindsight that that was okay. I don't think I was too harsh, but I did try to instill in them a sense that working hard is a good thing, and that if you have a talent, it's almost as though you have a duty to develop it, and not waste it. Also, I very much wanted all of my kids to have a sense of self-respect and to respect others. I think you get that from working to the best of your abilities and helping others, too. That's how I wanted them to conduct themselves, always.

It boils down to self-discipline. As a parent, I think you have to help your kids develop that. Sometimes they didn't like the rules we laid down, but I hope the rules helped them achieve goals in the long-run. For instance, I was strict about proper eating and early bedtimes before important games, and I never wavered from that rule. I remember young Brent being terribly disappointed when I wouldn't let him attend an important game of Wayne's one Saturday night at Maple Leaf Gardens in Toronto, because he had a hockey game of his own on Sunday. I just said, "You can't be up that late, you've got a game tomorrow . . . No, if you want to play hockey, then the night before, you're in bed early." There was no question in my mind, and the rule would have been the same if Wayne had a game the next day; he'd be in bed at a decent time. It was a ritual. I taught all the kids to pull their weight and not be a drag on the team.

Another thing I always told them: Listen to your coach! I'd teach them stuff in the backyard, and I might have had my own ideas sometimes about what would be the best thing to do out on the ice, but I was determined not to interfere. I didn't believe in hanging around during practices. It boils down to respect, once again.

My point, always, was that if you are going to do something, make sure you're focused, and do it right. I remember Glen coming home one time and saying to me, "Dad, I'm going to be an umpire this summer." I said, "You'll get that rule book, and you'll know every word in it, or you're not doing a thing." Well, that started it! Glen would be cocky and say, "Got the book right here, Dad, ask me anything you want." And I would start asking him all these complicated questions about the rules and what calls he'd have to make in various situations during a game. I really pushed him, and I was serious when I said, "If you don't know it, you're not doing it." Glen mastered that rule book.

BRENT GRETZKY: My dad used to say, "Enjoy life later, work for now. Train in the backyard, run, play baseball." There's that saying: "Kids in sports stay out of courts," and it's true. We never got into trouble. As for going to movies or hanging out at the mall, whatever, he'd say, "You can do all these things later in life." Dad's example was Wayne at the time. He would say, "Look at Wayne, he didn't go to movies on Friday nights with his friends. He would be outside training." So how could I say that didn't work?

Rest and proper eating, that was Dad's big thing. I remember being fourteen years old, playing Junior B. I'd be watching TV at nine o'clock at night, and he'd say, "Don't you have a game tomorrow? You should be in bed!" I'd have to go right to bed. We waited for Saturday nights to come, because we got to stay up late and watch the hockey game, the Leafs. He wasn't a drill sergeant about it, but he'd say, "If you want to play well, you should be resting." To this day, two nights before a game, he'll be saying to me, "Brent, you know, this is the most important night for rest, it's not just the night before."

We never argued with what my dad said. We'd want to go swimming in the hotel pools at the out-of-town tournaments, and he'd say no. I'd throw a fit, but he'd say, "It's because you use different muscles. How are you going to play tomorrow?" At the time, you don't really listen to it. You're a kid, you want to go. I look back on it today and think, "Wow, he was right." I thank him for those things now.

With all the kids' different involvements, there was a lot of juggling of responsibilities and activities. Still, I don't really know why I worried so much. It's just the way I was. I worried about my aging parents out at the farm, especially when my father became ill—he died in 1973. Then I worried about my mother being out there caring for Ellen and the farm all on her own. I worried about doing a good job at work and about having enough money to support my growing family. I worried through every hockey game my boys ever played. I worried about what was best for Wayne as his career unfolded at a very tender age and big, life-altering decisions had to be made, dealing with people I wasn't always sure I could trust. After he was launched, I worried about what was best for my other hockey-playing sons, Keith and Brent, who had their own challenges to face, coming up behind the Great Gretzky, with the same name on their sweaters and many expectations attached. When Glen was born with club feet, we were all devastated at first, wondering "why us?" I worried about making sure he got the best chance possible to correct the problem and have a normal life. Phyllis made many exhausting trips to the Hospital for Sick Children in Toronto, where Glen got excellent care. Thankfully, the surgery and physical therapy he had there were a success—when Glen wanted to play hockey, which, of course, he did, we made sure he got the skates he needed, too. But you can imagine how hard that was at the time, especially for Phyllis, contending with one child's health problems and raising four others as well.

PHYLLIS GRETZKY: It's just what you did in those days. You didn't think you were hard done by. I looked after the kids and house; Wally went to work and looked after the finances. I never had to write a cheque until after his stroke. Let's just say he wasn't what you would call a homebody or Mr. Fix-it. But he was on the go all the time, going out to the farm to help his mum, pruning the fruit trees and so on, taking the kids to their games. He'd make sure that rink in the backyard was clear, but our driveway would go unshovelled all winter. That does not happen now, with Wally taking care of our driveway and half our neighbours' as well! It makes us all laugh to think back on how it used to be. I remember there was a cement porch at the side of the house, with no railing. I wanted it down, but there was no way Wally was going to look after it. One Saturday, he was off with one of the kids—it was summertime, so it was probably a ball game with Wayne. We have a video of my brother-in-law Marvin and some other guys tearing it down with one of those jackhammers. It was better built and reinforced than they thought, and they needed a sledgehammer. But it was done by the time Wally got home.

He was always very concerned to see all the kids' games. Never sat down to eat, always on the fly doing something.

Stayed up late, catching up on things he wanted to do. He hardly ever missed a day of work. And that was tough, especially when he was travelling with Wayne. I'm not sure how we worked it all out. I would go to one kid's game and he'd go to another, sometimes we'd go together. But he'd work all day and go to a game at night, and then a tournament the next day, and maybe there was something that needed doing at the farm, working in the garden there, looking after Ellen. I'd be home with the kids. He'd run in between work and hockey games and ask for tea. I would fry him an egg and it would be stone-cold a half hour later when he finally ate it. He was just a whirlwind all the time.

Come winter, hockey was just what everybody in a town like Brantford did for recreation. I can't remember a time back then when there wasn't a bunch of kids out there together on the street or on the backyard rink, shooting a puck around, just getting out into the fresh air and having a great time. To me, that's what it's all about. There's the competitive aspect, sure, but some of the best friendships come from playing sports, as well. It's where kids can learn all kinds of things, about playing a game, about sportsmanship, team spirit, how to win and lose gracefully. How to have some discipline and pride in accomplishment and how to perfect a particular skill. And yes, how to just have fun! You don't have to win at all costs, or be the most talented player on the ice to enjoy a game. That's certainly how it was back when I was a kid, and what it was like at its best when my own kids were growing up. It bothers me sometimes that the emphasis has changed so much. Parents can be so aggressive when they watch their kids play a team sport at the beginning levels, I think they forget that the activity, whatever it may be, is supposed to be something their son or daughter enjoys doing, regardless of whether or not he or she is a superstar. I taught all my kids, and every kid I've ever coached, that if you have a good time, work hard and do your best, that is all that matters—and I really mean that

Of course, I don't deny that right from the beginning, I had a feeling my son Wayne might amount to something playing hockey, though I worried for awhile that, like me, he might be judged too small for the big leagues. That's why I always told him that if he couldn't be the biggest or fastest player, he could work on being the smartest. I wasn't the only one who saw that he was special, though. Lots of people who watched him play in Brantford as a kid had a hunch he was destined for greatness, or at least had the potential for it. You just don't see a kid with that kind of dedication and ability at such a young age very often. Mary and Sil next door used to say, "Wayne, you're going to make it to the NHL, and we're going to go to your first game." I'd just say, "I hope you're right." (The Rizzettos did come with us to see Wayne play his first game with the Indianapolis Racers.)

We've told this story so many times, it's legend for hockey fans now: Wayne could skate at the age of two, and we have the footage to prove it. Another thing people tease me about is how I used to be such a shutterbug. I always had cameras slung around my neck. I just got in the habit of taking pictures of Wayne and the other kids, whatever event they were participating in, and I'm glad I did (as are a few people who've published books on Wayne). It's a wonderful record to have, in light of all the achievements since. I even managed to get a shot of Wayne's first goal, at the age of six. He was pretty pleased with himself that day. He'd worked hard for it. But I don't suppose even I, as the proud dad of a talented and determined little player, had any idea what kind of amazing career that single, hard-won goal was inaugurating.

As well as a shutterbug, I was a pack rat—still am, actually, much to Phyllis's dismay. I saved everything, you name it: Wayne's first pair of skates, his first hockey sweater and stick, first trophy, all his other awards, newspaper stories and photos. And, of course, I liked to display all my kids' trophies and other mementos from their lives in sports. I hope I can say this without sounding boastful: we have a lot of trophies and memorabilia in our basement. Over the years, I've enjoyed showing it to people. I just love to see their faces when they come down and look at some of this stuff. I know it can brighten someone's day, especially a kid's, and that's made all the collecting worthwhile, right from the beginning. Don't forget, it's important not just from a sentimental point of view. As it turned out, it was hockey history in the making. Ron Ellis, head of the Hockey Hall of Fame—and a pretty good player with the Leafs in his day—tells me it's rare to have such a thorough record of a hockey star's early days. That alone makes it fairly unique, and I'm very pleased about that, too. Regardless of how well a kid ends up doing in sports, it's nice to have the mementos. And you never know when the Hall of Fame might come calling . . .

MURRAY ANGUS, FRIEND, CHARITY TOURNAMENT ORGANIZER: People always used to ask Wally, "Who's gonna be the next Wayne Gretzky?" Or they'd come up to him at a minor-league game and say, "This kid's the next Wayne Gretzky, don't you think?" Wally would always respond very politely, "Yeah well, he could very easily be, mmhmm, yep." Meanwhile, he was probably thinking, "Not likely." I remember I went over to the house once. Wayne was with the Oilers at the time, and Wally was sorting through home movies in the basement. He said to me, "Come here, you gotta watch this." It was Wayne skating around when he was about ten years old. And Wally said, "You wanna know who's gonna be the next Wayne Gretzky? The next ten-year-old kid you see who can do that!" One-handed stick stuff, you know. He's dodging and weaving in with these kids. His stick was like an extension of his arm.

When we got to our new home and as soon as I was up and about from my accident, I flooded our backyard to make a rink. Wayne spent most of his childhood winters out there and on the Nith River behind the old farmhouse, where I learned to skate myself. His grandmother Mary would sit in her chair in the living room and field his goals as he shot a plastic puck at her shins when he was just shin-high himself. It's no wonder she became his number-one fan. And never underestimate the power of a doting grandmother. I do like to tell people about the time when young Paul Reinhart (he and Wayne love this story, too), who was playing defence for Kitchener against Wayne's Brantford team back in the early '70s, checked Wayne into the boards. Grandma Mary was in the stands and didn't understand that Paul was just doing his job, that it was part of the game. She was so incensed, she marched right down from her seat and started clobbering Paul with her purse. I'm sure no one there will ever forget the sight, but it was the last time we let Wayne's grandmother sit by herself while watching a live game!

I used to take Wayne to my own hockey practices and games when he was just a toddler, and he'd sit there, keenly watching the action. Even back then, you could see there was a kind of intensity there. He took to the ice so naturally, I've often said, his life in hockey always seemed to be predestined. It's some kind of gift, there's no doubt about it. I always tell people who think I had something to do with his talent that making the rink was more self-preservation than anything else: Wayne loved skating so much, I'd freeze at the public outdoor rink or arena while he was doing what he loved best for literally hours on end. At least with the rink at home, I could be in the house staying warm!

Mary and Sil, whose son used to play out there too, had a bank of lights installed. Wayne would stay out till long after dark practicing his moves, shooting a puck around. Phyllis used to get a bit upset about it sometimes, urging me to bring him in and wondering what the neighbours would think of a family who let a six-year-old skate out there till ten at night. But that is what made Wayne happy, and we certainly never forced him or any of the others. That's why when parents ask Wayne to urge their children to practice as much as he did, he says, "I can't do that." Wayne did it because he loved it, not because someone told him he had to, and he doesn't believe kids get better when it's something they don't enjoy.

To tell you the truth, Wayne was good at most sports he tried, including lacrosse and long-distance running. And, as he's said himself, if you took his passion for hockey and doubled it, that's how he felt about baseball. He was quite a good little pitcher, even trained himself to be both right- and left-handed. When he was eleven, he played for the Chatham, Ontario, travelling team in the All-Canada Championships in Saskatchewan, and the team won. Who knows, if Wayne had been born and raised in the United States and had the right coaching, he might have ended up a pro baseball player instead. Personally, I'm glad he stuck with hockey.

CHARLIE HENRY, HOCKEY COACH, FAMILY FRIEND: I remember seeing Wayne play baseball in Brantford. He told me he would hit a home run to a particular spot near centre field, and he did. He called a shot, at fifteen years old. And he came down that dugout and grabbed me and said, "I told you I was gonna do it!" That, to me, just proved that there was nothing he couldn't do. And he didn't do it to be a hot dog. No, he wasn't a showman. Just to put himself under pressure. To say, "I'm gonna do it," and then do it. Oh, he was an excellent ball player. He loved ball. He played lacrosse, but he loved baseball more. He loved it. He knew all the stats and the players.

Meanwhile, our daughter, Kim, was turning into a terrific runner — obviously a chip off the old block there. She got involved in track and field and, in her early teens, won some provincial and eventually national titles. There was even talk among her coaches of grooming her for the Olympics. Unfortunately, Kim injured her ankle when she was fifteen and never pursued running after that.

While she was doing it, though, I did push her to eat right and keep herself in top form, because I saw the potential she had. I think at the time, she sometimes didn't like that I did that. My friend Charlie Henry from Ottawa tells me that when Kim went there to visit one summer, she wanted to run on the local track but asked if it was okay if she didn't stick to the diet and sleep routine I'd recommended. I suppose I was being a stickler, but I knew it was the only way for anyone to become a champion.

As Keith and Brent grew up, it became clear that they, too, had talent when it came to playing hockey. I can tell you, it was sometimes tough to juggle all their schedules, but Phyllis and I really did make an effort to get out and see as many of their games as possible, to encourage them and be there for them as much as we had with Wayne. We understood from an early time that with all the focus and media attention on Wayne—don't forget, that all began when he was just a little guy of six!—it would be possible for our other kids to feel neglected, and we did not want that.

BRENT: He got all of us skates at pretty much the same age: two or three years old. We were playing competitive hockey when we were five or six. We didn't miss a practice, and afterwards we'd come home and skate in the backyard. He'd come out with pylons and nets, and he'd videotape us and instruct us on how to skate, how to shoot. You know, he's the best coach we've ever had. Because we were his kids, he knew us better than anybody. Even in the pros, there's different ways to treat players. They can be yelled at or pampered. My dad knew how to relate to us. I don't think he showed any favouritism toward Wayne. He taught everyone the same thing—Wayne was just a heck of a lot better, the way he took it! Right after games, we'd go downstairs, watch the videotapes, and he'd point out what we were doing right. That was the main thing. With each child, my dad focused on what we did right and how to do it even better. He just wanted you to build on whatever you did best, whether it was skating or passing, whatever. He never put fighting into the backyard. His philosophy was, how do you expect to score if you're sitting in the penalty box?

I think he took a quote from a baseball player who said, "You never know who's going to be in the stands watching you." We tried to play with that in mind. And if my dad was in the stands—Whoooo! We tried our best!

KEITH GRETZKY: I kind of liked it when he didn't go to a game! I remember one game my mum came to, and afterwards, I said, "Mum, just tell Dad I played good." I had one goal and an assist. I didn't play very well. So Mum went home, and Dad asked, "How did he play?" She said, "Good." And then a few days later, he was waiting outside a practice, talking to some of the parents. And he came home and said to my mum, "What game did you go to? He played like a dog!" He'd heard from the other parents!

His big thing was rest, rest, rest. I remember, I was nineteen, in Junior A, I got traded from Belleville to Hamilton, and my coach said, "Oh great, you can live at home. It's only a twenty-minute drive." Usually you get billeted out. I lasted a week. I said, "I gotta get a billet! Dad wants me to go to bed at nine o clock! I'm nineteen!"

You see parents push their kids to live their dreams. I once ran a minor hockey rink in California, and I saw this all the time, and I thought, "Holy cow, they want their kid to be the next superstar in the NHL and yet my dad never would push us like that." That's the bad part of hockey now. People think that must be what he did, yet it's far from the truth. He got us involved in other things besides hockey, and although he pushed us to do well, we also knew it was up to us what we did with our lives.

I remember travelling with my friends John Mowat and Butch Steele to Brent's OHL games when he was with the Belleville Bulls. I'd finish a shift at work around mid-afternoon, Phyllis would make us a lunch for the road, and we'd pull out of the laneway around four in the afternoon. I'd fall asleep in the car until we got to Belleville. I'd wake up every once in awhile to say to whoever was driving, "Don't get a speeding ticket. But don't be late."

BUTCH STEELE: Before his aneurysm, the way Walter would watch a game his boys were in—he'd smoke a pack of cigarettes before the national anthem. He was a nervous wreck. If we went to Wayne's games, or young Brent's or Keith's, we'd pick up a quart of milk on the way there, because of his ulcer. Watching a game would get it going. We'd be home at three or four in the morning, and he'd be back to work by eight.

I always enjoyed watching Keith and Brent play hockey. They are both gifted athletes. But to compare them to Wayne is unfair. Compare them to other kids who play Major A, and we can have a discussion that would last for hours. My friend Bob Coyne remembers being involved with Brent when he was in Junior B, and always said Brent had "more moves than a rattlesnake." He could captivate an audience. He still can, playing in the United Hockey League, which is a pro league in the northeastern United States. He is an excellent skater, a good playmaker. Keith was very much an instinct player. He just knew where to be, all the time. He had great hands. Bob worked with him in hockey schools, and he's said to me, "The things Keith can do with a puck are just like . . . Whoa! Where'd you learn to do this, kid?" He was very, very good. But was he Wayne? No. Should he have been? NO! He was Keith. And he was a very good Keith, just as Brent is a very good Brent. This is the attitude we've had over the years. We tried to stress with our kids that everyone has something valuable to offer, and not everyone can be a superstar.

> BRENT: We knew there was going to be comparison between us and Wayne, but Dad would never get into that, because I guess then he'd be doing it, too. But in a roundabout way, he'd just say, "Do your best." Hockey was his life. He wanted to be with Wayne every game, and I think with every other boy, same thing goes. When he went to my games, he would stand in the corner and videotape, and if I was playing bad, he would kind of look at me, and I knew I had to pull up my socks.

CHARLIE HENRY: You know, over the years, we've seen Brent play in the minors, we've seen Keith play in the minors, like we went to see Wayne. I remember one time travelling fifteen hours with Wally to see Keith play. He made sure he saw everybody. He tried to help the other guys to play in the NHL, to play pro. And there was a lot of pressure on those kids. I can remember when they came into the Ontario league. It wasn't them people saw, it was the name. It was hard to have that name on the sweater. And they were great hockey players. If they had had any other name, they might have been better treated. People expected so much. It put them in the limelight right away. And often it takes time for a player to become exceptional. They didn't get the benefit of the doubt there. But on the other hand, Wayne—there was nothing he didn't do for his kid brothers. He knew what they were going through. He was always so good to them. It wasn't his fault.

Some people have tried to suggest from time to time that there's bad feelings between Wayne and his brothers, but that's absolutely not true. Keith and Brent love their older brother, and he loves them. Wayne's always been a terrific fan and supporter of his younger brothers and sister; Charlie's right, there's nothing he wouldn't do for them.

But there was no denying that Wayne had something extra special going for him in the hockey department, and right from the beginning, I was prepared to nurture that along in whatever way I could. Although the minor hockey rules said he couldn't join a novice team at the age of six, I took him to the tryout anyway, and he made the team, just because of his adept stick handling. He was a proud number eleven, but he was so much smaller than the other players, he really stood out. His sweater hung so low, he had to tuck it into the back of his pants and, as every hockey fan knows, that became a trademark for him.

Wayne scored only one goal that year (the one I managed to capture on camera), and he didn't win any awards. I could tell he was not happy about that, and I remember saying to him, "Don't worry about it, son. If you keep working at this, one day you'll have so many, you won't know what to do with them." Years later, when Wayne brought home the Stanley Cup and received the Order of Canada . . . it's hard to describe the feeling.

After that first year of working to keep up with the bigger kids, Wayne won his first trophy: the Wally Bauer Award for being the most improved Novice all-star player during the Brantford Minor Hockey Association's 1968–69 season. As has been well documented over the years, there really was no stopping him after that. He went from one goal in his first year to twenty-seven the next. Four years later, by the age of ten, he went from 196 goals the year before to a stunning 378. That's really when the media picked up on the story of "the kid from Brantford" big time, and Wayne was interviewed by newspapers and on radio and TV shows across the country.

Being "the one to watch" was tough for Wayne, because he was a shy kid, or at least kind of like me back then, more reserved in personality. We often recall the story of the hockey banquet where he met his idol, Gordie Howe, for the first time. It's where the famous picture was taken of the two of them, when Wayne was ten.

They're both smiling away, and Gordie's got a hockey stick around Wayne's neck. They hit it off, but there was a mix-up with the announcer, who introduced Wayne as a speaker. The poor kid had no speech prepared. He stood up and stared at the hundreds of people out there in front of the head table, and was literally speechless. It was Gordie who rescued him. He just walked over and said, "I think anyone who just scored that many goals doesn't have to make a speech." Everyone applauded, and Wayne got to sit down. That was the beginning of a connection between those two that carries on to this day. I'm sure Gordie knew back then that this kid might one day surpass his own achievements in hockey.

We travelled around the country to watch Wayne play. By the time he was thirteen, he had gained so much attention, he had been all over Canada and had an agent. Meanwhile, at home in Brantford, eleven-year-old Kim was into her track and field in a big way, travelling to meets around the province, and winning a lot of races, eventually proving herself to be "one to watch" at the national level. It was too soon to tell just what kind of player Keith would be, but he was forging his own way in minor hockey; Glen, at age five, was proving to be a smart and active kid, nicely overcoming all the difficulties with his feet and keen to get into his own pair of skates. Baby Brent, bringing up the rear, was showing signs he'd soon be toddling toward the hockey arena himself. Despite all of Wayne's successes on the rink and the attention he was gaining far and wide, we still wanted him to have as normal a family life as possible and to work hard at school, which he did—he managed to be an A student, too.

WAYNE: People might not believe it, but although my father's biggest passion—apart from fishing and photography—was seeing his sons do well in hockey, he wasn't motivated by money. That just didn't enter his mind. That's why he has a hard time fathoming the way it is with some hockey parents today. I mean, hockey was the focus of his life, but every Sunday morning he got us up for church. I never missed church for the first fifteen years of my life. He didn't even go regularly himself until 1980, but he made sure we went. The nice thing is that now when I go to Brantford, we go to church as a family, and I see the same people there as I did when I was a kid. That's just incredible to me.

In April, 1974, Wayne recorded his one thousandth minor hockey goal. People could see he had the potential to do things in hockey that no one had ever done before. Still, with all the success came pressure for Wayne, and there was resistance and skepticism among some spectators and reporters. Wayne was aware of that and always tried to rise to the challenge of performing to the best of his abilities and proving people wrong.

I remember how it was when I first met Charlie Henry, who would become a lifelong close friend. We were in Belleville, watching Wayne play, and Wayne was wearing these white gloves. I overheard Charlie making a remark along the lines of, "Could he skate in the dark in the white gloves," and everyone around chuckled. It's true, they were so bright, they practically glowed. I knew people assumed that Wayne was trying to show off and draw attention his way. I thought it wouldn't hurt to introduce myself to this wisecracker. I guess Charlie felt a little embarrassed. He said, "Hey, nothing wrong with the kid. He's a great player." Later, I told Charlie the truth about those gloves. The Cooper company, now Bauer, had sent them to the sporting goods store in Brantford especially for Wayne. But the owner knew I wouldn't just take them. So he said he'd give them to me for ten bucks, which I thought was a good deal. Wayne wore them not only because he liked them, but because he knew we didn't have a lot of money to throw around. It might have been the first product endorsement Wayne was asked to do, but it certainly wasn't his last. These companies had good reason to suppose they were on to a good thing.

Wayne had a lot of enthusiastic supporters in those days, people like Eddie Ramer, Bryan Wilson and Charlie Henry, who we have always appreciated and who are dear friends to this day. We got to know Eddie when Wayne was ten. He started following Wayne's progress when he was about eight or nine years old, when he was still playing hockey for the young Nadrosky Steelers. Eddie was among those who seemed to know right away that he was seeing someone special. So he made a point of going to a lot of the games. In Wayne's last year of Peewee, Eddie felt he was going to have his most prolific scoring year and he decided he would keep stats on every game. He didn't know our family at the time, he just enjoyed watching Wayne play. That was the year Wayne became famous for scoring 378 goals. So Eddie had this chart drawn up and decided he would present it to us. He phoned up and told me that he had something to give to Wayne and me, honouring that particular year. When he came over with it, we were pretty overwhelmed by such a generous gesture. Today, Eddie's chart is one of the first things you see in the display cases of the Gretzky exhibit at the Hockey Hall of Fame. We were truly touched when people showed that kind of interest in our son.

Mostly, the kids Wayne played with didn't have a problem with him. But some of the other hockey parents and people in the media weren't that fond of him. There was a lot of naysaying. Many just assumed he was a flash in the pan, an arrogant show-off with a pushy parent who got him more ice time than he deserved. In fact, because he was so good at all the sports he played, he got that kind of response whether it was lacrosse or baseball or distance running. Some people just seemed to have a problem with a kid who was that talented.

The truth was, although Wayne loved to score as much as the next guy and didn't hide his pride when he did, with that famous kick of his, he was always a team player. He looked out for the other guy right from the youngest age. I recall one time before a game, during that season when he scored 378 goals, he came to me and said, "Dad, there's a boy on the team, I feel so sorry for him, he hasn't scored a single goal. You watch, Dad, tonight I'm going to help him score a goal." And he did that. He was ten years old, the top scorer, and yet he set up a play so that his teammate could finally score a goal.

It was a long time ago, and frankly I don't feel any anger any more about the negative attitudes some people had toward Wayne. A little while back, I was out at the arena with my friend Warren MacGregor. One of the parents who was really among the worst for verbally abusing Wayne out on the ice in those days came up and shook my hand, all smiling and friendly, asking me how I was doing. Afterwards, Warren said to me, "Wally, how can you talk to that man after the way he used to behave?" But I say, what's the point of holding a grudge? It's over, move on.

In some ways, I could understand how people felt. You're a parent, you've got a kid out there who you want to have as much ice time as possible, and you see this other kid who just seems to score all the goals and get all the attention. It got so bad, some people actually booed when Wayne came out on the ice. I guess they never stopped to think what kind of effect that could have on a young player. He might have been talented beyond his years, but he was just a little boy. After a game where there'd been a lot of abuse from other parents, he'd come home and spend the night crying in his room. Looking at it from a kid's perspective, it must have been confusing: you go out on the ice, give your best effort for the love of the game, and you get booed? It hurt him, and it hurt Phyllis and me to see him so upset.

We could see how the atmosphere of resentment in our hometown was affecting Wayne, and that led us to make the tough decision to send him to Toronto to live and play hockey when he was just fourteen years old. A friend called and asked if Wayne would like to play on a team in Toronto, go to high school there and live with the family of a teammate. Wayne was eager to go, but as parents, we really did not want to see that happen. Added to my worries was the thought of the kind of trouble a young teenager could get into in the big city, living away from his parents. It was the early '70s, and we were, of course, worried about drugs. I remember arguing with him about it, and finally Wayne said, "Dad, you're worried about me getting into drugs in Toronto. Just name the drugs and give me a few hours. I'll just go over to the high school here in Brantford and bring some home." I saw the point he was making. Reluctantly, Phyllis and I said yes, he could go.

It was a turning point in his life and the life of our family, because he never lived at home again. But we worked hard to remain close and to provide all the support we could for Wayne, even if it was at a distance. As much as possible, he visited us and we visited him and went to see as many of his games as we could. Talking on the phone late at night, when the long-distance rates were lowest, became part of our way of life, and large phone bills became part of our budget! But any fears and worries we had were put to rest. We were very fortunate to find a good family for Wayne to live with in Toronto, Bill and Rita Cornish. I think he was probably lonely sometimes, aware of how much his abilities in hockey were setting him aside from the rest of the kids his age, but he could go to school like a normal kid, play hockey in the evenings and on weekends, and enjoy a bit of anonymity, the last in his life really, in a bigger city. He was supposed to play Bantam at that age, but he was good enough for Junior A and so ended up on the Toronto Young Nationals, playing with young men who were much larger than he was. I'd always told him his strength would be his brains, not his size, and that continued to be the case.

With four kids still at home, family life continued to centre around sports: hockey tournaments, track meets, baseball games. Wayne maintained a good relationship with his siblings, even if he didn't get to see them as much as we'd all have liked. In 1977, despite our initial misgivings about Wayne going even further away, he was drafted to the Sault Ste. Marie Greyhounds. But that turned out well, too, and it's where he first wore the number ninety-nine.

We couldn't always get to those games, of course, but my friend Bryan Wilson and I figured out a way to be part of the action all the way down in Brantford.

BRYAN WILSON: Wally and I, we had this thing built. It was two pieces of wood from a crate, like a pyramid with a wire in it as an aerial, and we'd plug it into the portable radio and listen to the Sault Ste. Marie games. He'd be sitting at one end of the table, I'd be at the other. There was only one earphone we had to share. And I'd say, "Wally, what do you hear?" He'd say, "I think he just scored." And I'd be saying, "Well, let me hear!" And, of course, he would hardly let me listen to the game! I'd get so mad. I'd have to make the tea. I'd say, "Wally, I've made three pots already, I haven't listened to anything, because you're the only one with the earphone!" It was funny, the two of us sitting at the table. Oh, we listened to almost every game that Sault Ste. Marie played. Or at least Wally did!

I must have smoked a lot of cigarettes and coated my poor old stomach with a lot of milk around the time when Wayne was getting ready to join the pro leagues. He was under age, of course, and that didn't sit well with the NHL. His agent, Gus Badali, thought it was best to go for the World Hockey Association (WHA), and, once again, that decision turned out for the best. A few deals fell through, but, in the end, it looked like a guy by the name of Nelson Skalbania was pretty serious about Wayne. Skalbania flew him, Phyllis and me out to Vancouver to meet with him. It was pretty funny; I'll never forget him picking us up at the airport in a Rolls Royce. It might as well have been a jalopy, because it smoked all the way back to Skalbania's house. He advised me, "Walter, never buy a Rolls Royce," and I can honestly say to this day I never have.

When Wayne signed that deal, his first large professional contract, we were all pretty relieved, even though it wasn't clear yet where he was going to play. It ended up being in Indianapolis, with the Racers. It wasn't a great season. People weren't all that interested in the team, or in Wayne, and Skalbania was losing money. After only eight games, he decided Wayne should move, and Gus Badali advised Wayne to pick Edmonton, where the WHA was attracting more attention and the team was more likely to be bought by the NHL.

And that of course, was the beginning of a whole new era for Wayne, and for hockey, and in a lot of ways, for me and the family, too. It had always been exciting being Wayne's dad, but as the '80s got started, I don't think any of us could have dreamed about what life was going to be like now, with a bona fide NHL star on board.

Every hockey parent of a kid with a little talent dreams of him making it to the NHL. All the hard work of so many years was paying off, but it sure didn't stop just because Wayne had "made it." Far from it! Not that we'd have it any other way. I can only say that even though it was a dream come true, for Wayne, for me, for all of us, it wasn't always what we expected it to be, either. But if nothing else, the Gretzky family of Varadi Drive, Brantford, Ontario, Canada, knew how to rise to a challenge. The "fame and glory" might have thrown us for a loop sometimes, but one thing was for sure—life was never going to be dull!

chapter three

"PINCH ME, MY SON'S IN THE NHL"

So many books have been written about Wayne. There are dozens, by now, that detail his achievements as the NHL star who spent his career shattering every record in sight. Anyone with his kind of success and fame is bound to generate a lot of curiosity in the public. People marvel at his performances on the ice, but they also want to know what it was like behind the scenes during those golden years. What's it been like to be Wayne's dad?

Wayne's celebrity didn't come upon him, or us, suddenly. Don't forget, people were paying close attention to him, in both positive and negative ways, from the time he was a kid in the minor leagues, outscoring his teammates and opponents—most often, boys who were older and bigger than him. Because there was a lot of jealousy toward him and my other boys when they were growing up, I would tell them to not only play their best every night, but also to cheer their teammates on. Have manners, be polite. Wayne was signing autographs in his teens, and one thing I did try to teach him was to appreciate his fans and treat them nicely. And I taught him and the other boys that when it came to the press, I expected them to tell the truth and not run away. If someone wanted to do an interview, I told them to try to do it. Take the time and talk to them.

I believe in being open, but still, you do have to wonder sometimes at the lengths to which people will go just to get near or collect some kind of souvenir of a famous person like Wayne. For awhile there, I was actually a little concerned about my younger kids walking home from school alone or being out on their own late at night. Like any parent, I was worried about what could happen to them, but especially once they had such a famous brother. I warned them to be careful and aware at all times, and, fortunately, nothing bad ever happened.

Being asked for autographs and mementos was one of the first indicators that things were going to be different now, for all of us, and by the '80s, such requests were a part of our life. We weren't the only ones who Wayne's fans would approach. Once Wayne really got going with the Oilers, even our extended family and friends started to get calls, out of the blue, from collectors and memorabilia hounds from all over the world, asking if they had any items of

Wayne's that they might like to sell. You can be sure that in the case of our true friends, the answer was and is no. Wayne has signed and given away things to family and friends, which they consider to be very special, beyond any mere monetary value.

We've even had people going through our garbage—honestly! I have to thank our neighbours for being so tolerant. Cars come through here all the time, clearly on the lookout for the Gretzky house, and often the people in the cars will stop and ask one of our neighbours, "Where's the Gretzkys'?" People get out and take photographs. It felt odd the first time a stranger knocked on our door and asked me to come out and pose for a picture, but I'm used to it by now.

Once, I was sitting in the living room, where I could see out the front window. Along came a car, which slowed down—obviously, it was someone coming to see the house where Wayne Gretzky grew up. Nothing unusual about that. Suddenly, the car doors flew open, and two young girls, around eleven or twelve, jumped out and ran onto the lawn. They bent down and started pulling up the grass! When they had a few clumps, they raced back to the car, and it sped off down the street. I just shook my head, amazed that anyone would want a piece of Gretzky grass. It was truly bizarre.

The funny thing is, a couple of years ago, I told that story during a speech in Kitchener, Ontario, and got a lot of laughs. A while later, I was at a Hallmark store, signing autographs and figurines of Wayne, and a lady came up and said, "Remember that story you told not long ago in Kitchener, about those two girls snatching the grass from your lawn? Well, I was the driver of the car." I couldn't believe it! I asked her whatever became of the girls, and she told me they were the daughters of family friends from Nova Scotia, who had been visiting her during summer holidays. Both girls were now grown up, still living in the east, married, with children of their own.

I was delighted to hear this, and I had an idea. I asked the woman if she'd give me their addresses, and she did. I went home, pulled up some grass and sealed it up in two plastic bags. I sent them off with two notes saying, "I imagine that grass you took is getting awfully old and dry. Here's some fresh grass. Yours truly, Walter Gretzky." You know, I never did hear back from them, but I get such a kick just thinking about the looks on their faces when they opened their packages and read those notes!

Being in the spotlight sure brought a lot of craziness to our lives, but, as I've mentioned, we had some time to get used to it. The younger members of the family can't remember a time when Wayne wasn't getting a lot of attention. You never knew how a person might react to Wayne or even to you, just because you were related to him. On the up side were all the people who recognized exceptional ability when they saw it. They sincerely wanted to see Wayne realize his potential and were excited by the possibilities. On the down side were his critics, who either resented his talent or thought it was too good to be true.

One person in the media who always criticized Wayne, and I could never figure out why, was sportscaster Dick Beddoes. It didn't matter what Wayne did, Beddoes just always kept saying that Wayne was overrated, that he wasn't as talented as everyone thought, that eventually his luck would run out and he'd fade away into oblivion. It was hard to figure out why the man had such a negative attitude. But years later, I was talking about him with one of the local sportscasters who said, "No, Walter, Dick didn't really believe that Wayne was that bad. In fact, he had a lot of respect and admiration for him. He just kept saying all those nasty, outrageous things to keep his ratings up."

Think about it: more people would tune in if Dick Beddoes made controversial statements than if he just stuck with more predictable comments. That had never occurred to me.

I was often taken aback by what people had to say about Wayne. I'll never forget the day back in 1989 when I was flying to Edmonton to see him break Gordie Howe's scoring record, as we knew he likely would at the game that night. It was all very nice on the plane, since Wayne had decided to bring me out first-class. Making conversation, I asked the lady sitting next to me where she was going, then realized that was kind of a stupid question, since we were on a plane, going to the same place. She said she was going to visit her daughter, who she hadn't seen since her wedding several months earlier. She asked what I was doing, and I said I was going to see my son. Then I pulled a magazine out of the bin in front of me and, wouldn't you know, it was the *Sports Illustrated* with Wayne on the cover as Athlete of the Year. The lady started in, "Oh that Wayne Gretzky, he's no good." She proceeded to criticize him for the next few minutes. She really had nothing positive to say about him at all. I should have told her right then and there who I was, but I didn't want to embarrass her. I just put the magazine back in its place, with the cover facing in, and tried to avoid conversation.

Soon the flight attendant came along to ask us all what we wanted to drink with our breakfasts. She went along the row, addressing us by name. "And what will you be having, Mrs. Smith? And Mrs. Jones?" Finally, she got to me. I was cringing as she said, "And Mr. Gretzky, I guess you're going out to Edmonton to see Wayne score that goal? You must be very proud of your son." Well, the look on that lady's face! I felt sorry for her, but, on the other hand, I guess she had it coming. She hardly touched her breakfast, just sipped at her coffee, and I had trouble eating the food in front of me, too. I'll tell you, it was a very silent flight. We just sat side by side, our arms crossed over our chests, staring straight ahead the entire time.

People have often wondered why I didn't retire when Wayne hit the big leagues. I remember that when I worked for Bell Canada, I used to dream all the time about the day I'd retire. Although juggling Wayne's travel schedule with my job wasn't something I complained about, and I was able to use my vacation days to go to the boys' tournaments over the years, it all would have been easier if I'd had more leisure time and flexibility. I would think, "When I retire, I'll be able to sleep in if I want to, stay up late, go away for two or three days at a minute's notice and not have to worry about getting back." Of course, the irony is, only a few months after I did finally retire, I had the stroke, and that cured me of making plans and dreaming too far into the future for the rest of my life!

I did, at one point during those years, take a six-month leave of absence, but as much as I might have fantasized about the freedom of leaving my job, I didn't feel ready. Wayne kept urging me to give it up for good. His thinking was that I could do some work for him. I guess in the end I felt better earning my own money, living in a house I bought and paid for myself. It was a matter of self-respect. Also, what kind of example would I be setting for my other kids, who were still either living at home or just leaving the nest, if I quit my job and lived off someone else's success? That's not a very good lesson on how to live your life, in my opinion. You have to make your own way, and I wanted my kids to understand that.

After the six months were up, I had to decide by eight o'clock on the morning of the day I was due back whether I'd work or be done with it. The night before, I sat around for a long time thinking about what I should do. Phyllis had already gone to bed. Finally, I went in to the bedroom and said, "Phyllis, wake me up in the morning. I don't want to be late, I'm going to work." I'm glad I did. I put in my thirty-four years, and I have a pension from Bell Canada. Mind you, I never see it, because Phyllis spends it, but, all joking aside, I'm happy I went back.

I know my stubborn independent attitude was frustrating for Wayne sometimes. He wanted to give us a new house on a couple of occasions, but we didn't feel right about it. The first place he bought for us was huge, a mansion. We went and looked, but we just could not see living there—it wasn't us. Next, he tried to surprise us by buying a property that he thought we could build something on. That plan got foiled when I was at city hall one day and a woman in the planning department, who obviously did not realize it was a secret, asked me about the property. Again, Phyllis and I said no to uprooting ourselves. It's not that we didn't appreciate the gestures. I'm proud of the fact that Wayne is a generous-hearted person, always thinking of other people and eager to share his good fortune. The crazy thing is, once he became a star and could really afford anything he wanted, people started giving him things: cars, trips, watches, works of art, you name it. That's the strange way celebrity works. You have to have a good head on your shoulders to handle it, especially in the beginning. I think Wayne has managed really well to keep all the consequences of fame and wealth in perspective.

He has helped the family, too, no doubt about it. We finally put an addition on our home, which really comes in handy with a family the size of ours, especially now that our grandchildren are coming along. And Wayne's wife, Janet, insisted on giving us a pool in the backyard, where the rink used to be. We've been here forty years and we're very comfortable. We don't plan on moving any time soon.

While I was happy to continue working for Bell, I must admit that once Wayne became famous, I sometimes ended up in awkward situations on the job—even worse than that encounter with the lady on the airplane. On one occasion, I arrived at an office to fix a teleprinter, and the young woman at the receptionist's desk asked me where I was from.

"Brantford," I told her.

"Oh, so do you know Wayne Gretzky?" Not wanting to get into it or seem boastful, I just said, "Yeah, sure, everybody knows everybody in Brantford."

Well, she proceeded to launch into a scathing attack on my

son, how her fiancé had played with him in minor hockey, and how Wayne was nothing but an overhyped so-and-so who didn't deserve all the attention he got. She was really quite vicious in her remarks. I was under the desk repairing a wire, just praying she'd stop and that she wouldn't expect me to respond to what she was saying. Mostly, though, I wanted to stick close to the phone on the desk, because I was expecting a call from another Bell man, who would be checking to see if the repair had worked.

When I turned away for just a moment, the phone rang and the young woman picked it up. After a couple of seconds, her eyes got wide and she gasped. I swear, she threw down the receiver and backed away from the desk and out of the office. "You're NOT . . . !" she kept saying, "You're NOT . . . !"

Of course, my colleague had asked if he could speak to Mr. Gretzky.

I have to admit, I felt sorry for her. Funnily enough, I never again got a call to do a repair job at that office. Incidents like that taught me over the years that whenever the subject of Wayne came up, even if I sounded like I was boasting, it was best for everybody concerned if I just immediately jumped in and said, "I'm his dad, you know!"

I may have kept my day job, but that didn't stop me from following Wayne's career closely. I'll admit, I got quite wound up when it came to hockey, especially if it was a game in which a son of mine happened to be playing. If I was watching a game on TV, I would get really upset if the people around me talked too much. A few friends used to come by regularly to watch a game in the basement with me: Butch, Eddie, Bryan and Ronnie Finucan. I'm afraid they'd all tell you, I could be grouchy if they didn't keep quiet. It got so bad, and Phyllis got so fed up with me, that we ended up having two TVs in different rooms, so anyone who thought they had to chat while watching the game could watch it elsewhere.

> BRENT: You didn't make noise while Dad was watching the game on TV. No way! He had his own room, and we were the rowdy crowd in the other room: me, Glen, my mum, a couple of our friends. Glen used to put signs up for the playoffs, like seat designations, banners.
>
> My dad had just a plain room. He'd be watching TV with a red phone right beside the couch, so he could pretend he was calling Glen Sather to give him some coaching tips. You had to be quiet if you went in to his room—there were no ifs, ands or buts about it. If you got too loud, he'd look at you and you just knew: shut up and get out.

I have to thank our neighbour down the street, Roly Bye, who installs satellite dishes for a living, for making it possible for us to watch a good number of Wayne's games that we'd otherwise have missed. We got to know Roly in the late '80s. Wayne had already given us a dish so we could watch all his western games— it certainly beat an old radio rig-up with one little earphone!—but the thing wasn't very reliable. I phoned Roly one day and said, "Wayne's playing tonight, and I can't get a darn channel on this dish. Do you think you could come up and look at it for us?" He fooled around with it and managed to get a picture, but it was terrible and there was no sound at all. He didn't think there was much hope of getting what he needed to fix it that day, but he kindly said, "Walter, if you want to come down to the house tonight, we'll be watching the game there. And you're welcome to bring your friends." I didn't want to impose, but I didn't want to miss the game, either.

> ROLY BYE: That's a night I won't forget. I didn't think Walter was going to make it, you know. The starting time was eight o'clock. I thought he'd be here early, but just about right on the button, the door flies open, and in comes Wally. He sat on the chesterfield, my wife, Gloria, sat in her chair and I sat beside him. I said, "Do you want a beer, Wally?" He said, "Oh no, I can't drink beer." "Pop?" "No, I've got ulcers. I can drink milk, though." So I got him a big glass of milk. I've never seen a guy so intense. You wouldn't believe it. He sat there like a little kid with his feet under him. And he was like that right until they got about three goals ahead. Then he just laid back and relaxed, put his feet on the coffee table.

Thanks to Roly, we saw all of Wayne's games. If there was a problem with the reception, he'd come over on those cold winter nights to fix it. Sometimes he was already in his pyjamas, but he never complained. We would stay up till three in the morning, watching the game. It was a way of life around here!

EDDIE RAMER: Watching Wayne's games with Edmonton, on television, Walter'd have his watch out, seeing how much ice time Wayne was getting, and he could get very upset: "He's not out there for the power play! Why isn't he out there?!" or "They took him off before the power play finished!" Very intense. Enjoyed it thoroughly, but was right into it.

BUTCH STEELE: Oh, he would pace and pace and pace. He would just be stomach and nerves and smoking and pacing. Back and forth. And whether it was Wayne or Keith or Brent, it didn't matter which one of the boys, if they had a key game, if they didn't play well, you know, he wouldn't get upset, but he'd say, you could have done this better or that.

People joke about me being harsh on the boys about their performances. I do recall times when Wayne would score five of eight goals in the game, and I'd say, well, why didn't you score all eight? And when he called me after one game and said, "I did it, Dad, I did it!" I said, "Did what?" "I broke the record!" And I said, "What took you so long?" But really, of course, I was proud of him. In fact, I'll say the thing that made me proudest was the fact that he'd take the time after a victory to call his dad and tell him about it. Being thoughtful like that is one of his greatest achievements, in my opinion.

WAYNE: What can I say? My dad was there every step of the way for me, so it was just the most natural thing in the world for me to think of and include him whenever something major happened. Those were special times, and I knew how much it meant to him to see me, to see all of us, succeed.

I do believe in gentlemanly conduct and helping others out whenever you can, even if it means going a little out of your way. Bob Coyne teases me about this. We started to get to know each other in the late '80s, when he was taking a Brantford minor hockey team to Sweden. I called Bob three or four weeks ahead of when they were scheduled to leave, which was on Boxing Day. I said, "Bob, if you're taking a team of kids to Sweden, you'll need some of Wayne's stuff to trade over there. European kids are big on trading at tournaments. I've got lots of stuff; you'll want to come up here and get some." Bob tells me now that he just didn't have the nerve to come pounding on our door to take me up on my offer. Two weeks went by, and I called him again. "You haven't come up," I said. "No, I've been busy." I said, "Well, get right up here. I've got all this stuff out. It's sitting here." He said, "When would you like me to come?" I said, "Tomorrow at four." Well, we missed that time for one reason or another, and we arranged for another date, and another date after that, but we didn't connect. And now we were down to Christmas night, and I called again. "Bob. Walter Gretzky. You still haven't got here." He said, "Well, it's Christmas night. We're flying out tomorrow morning." I said, "Get up here right now." He said, "I can't come to your house on Christmas, Walter. You have your whole family there and everything." I said, "No, no, no. They've all gone. It's quiet. Just Phyllis and me here right now. Come on up." So reluctantly he came up. Damn good thing. I had three green garbage bags full of

Wayne memorabilia. Everything from eight-by-tens to water bot-
tles with pictures of Wayne on them, buttons and pins. Phyllis
was happy to part with the pile, I'll tell you.

BOB COYNE: Now the problem was, how was I going to get
to Europe with this stuff? We went to the airport with these
garbage bags, and the security people looked at us and said,
"And WHAT is this?" I said, "Well, that's from Walter
Gretzky for kids to trade when they get to Europe, at the
hockey tournament." And as I was saying that, the pilot heard
me and came walking up. He said, "That's from Walter
Gretzky?" I said, "Yes." And he said, "I'll look after it." Not
another word was exchanged. The three bags disappeared.
Later in the flight, the pilot invited the kids up to see the
cabin, and I noticed, tucked in right behind him, on this 747,
three green garbage bags, full of Wayne paraphernalia.

You see, I believe things have a way of working out!

I enjoyed doing special stuff like that for kids, but the main
focus, always, was hockey. It's true that Wayne and I would discuss
the games in great detail, by phone or, if I'd been at a game, in
person afterwards. He even called me between periods. Wayne was
as intense about playing hockey as I was watching it. You'd see
him on the bench there during the game, beside the other players,
and you might see some of them chatting with each other, or looking down or away from the ice. Not Wayne. He would be watching the play non-stop. You'd see his head going back and forth, all
the time. He'd be looking at all the other players, sizing up their

moves and strategies, seeing if he could pick out weaknesses in the defensive line, if someone wasn't turning well in a certain direction or had a problem with their leg, that sort of thing.

CHARLIE HENRY: Walter was always an adviser to Wayne, and Wayne liked it when his dad was there. He'd call me and say, "Charlie, pick up my dad and come to the game. I'd have to get myself from Ottawa to Toronto, and then we'd be off to Chicago or someplace. Phyllis would drive Wally to the airport. Oh, Wally would be a nervous wreck during the game. He'd comment. He'd analyze Wayne and everybody else, too. But he's not loud. And if he had a criticism of someone and he met the player's parent afterwards, he'd be very nice. He'd say, "Your son played so well." And he meant it. Because at that level, you would have to be a pretty good athlete, just to be there. He was very gracious to everybody.

MURRAY ANGUS: I'd tag along with these guys to hockey games in Toronto or Detroit, Buffalo, Chicago. Listening to Walter and Wayne after a hockey game was incredible. These guys would talk this cryptic kind of language. Wally would say, "Well, you know, that shot in the second period . . ." and Wayne would reply, "Well, yeah, Kevin was coming up the side, and so-and-so was behind me and Messier was over here, and this guy was there, the goalie was going down, I had to shoot high." And Walter would say, "No, if you'd gone over there and left your stick down . . ." and they'd talk this way, Wayne a half sentence and Wally the other half. It was this whole amazing dialogue. You talk about two guys talking hockey! You realized they spoke the exact same hockey language. I don't mean the terms. I mean, Wally would say, "When you were coming in on that wing," and Wayne would know exactly what he was talking about, which play, say, in the middle of the second period. Those four seconds out of a whole hockey game. And Wayne would know because when he'd done it, he'd been totally aware that Wally would be thinking that he should have been over there instead.

As Wayne's celebrity grew, I did what I could to offer guidance and advice that I thought would help him stay grounded. But by the late '80s, after years of really intense work as an athlete and being in the spotlight, I knew Wayne was feeling stressed. He was being pulled in a lot of different directions. He'd get mobbed by fans wherever he went. He was dating Janet, who was a Hollywood actress, and the tabloid press was showing an intense interest in his personal life. I know he just wanted to hide sometimes. I think he always knew we were rooting for him here in Brantford, and that we were delighted whenever we got a chance to see him play and to get together after the games. We were even more delighted when he was able to be with us at home. If he sometimes felt overwhelmed by all the demands, surrounded as he was by agents, owners, lawyers and whoever else wanted a piece of him at any given time, I think he also knew that I was just a phone call away, and I'd always try to give him the only advice I thought made any sense: mainly, be genuine and keep it simple.

WAYNE: My father was my sounding board, whether it was about playing hockey or whatever else was going on for me. He was there all the time, and you just knew that his advice was the best advice you were going to get. I mean, he was my dad. Nobody knew me or the game of hockey better than he did.

Of course, we always wanted the best for him and were so happy when he did well in Edmonton and later in Los Angeles. People would often ask me to comment on Wayne's career during that period, especially on the deal Peter Pocklington made with Bruce McNall to trade him to the L.A. Kings. I suppose in the beginning, like so many other hockey fans, I was reluctant to see Wayne leave such a successful team as the Oilers, and even more reluctant to see him leave Canada. You knew it was the end of an era in lots of ways. It was no wonder that everyone, including Wayne, was very emotional about it at the time. But even though the decision might have been painful, everyone knew Wayne was going to be traded at some point, and I think he did the right thing in retaining his right to choose where he'd go, and in making the decision to go where he figured it made the most sense for him and Janet to base themselves and the family they planned to raise.

Quite frankly, I thought at first he'd be better off going to Detroit than Los Angeles and told him that. The team was more established and familiar to me, and closer to home. L.A. seemed like another planet, and I was a bit suspicious of the whole idea. For a while there, Wayne was pretty scared and worried about what his next move should be, because he was inclined to go with L.A. and knew I wasn't immediately behind that. But I spent a few days out there visiting Wayne, meeting with Bruce McNall, who I got to know and respect, and I changed my mind. I said to Wayne, "You know, maybe this would be the best place for you." I have to say it worked out pretty well for Wayne.

We're delighted that he and Janet have four great, healthy kids, and we always enjoy visiting them, even though L.A. is a long way from Brantford, in more ways than one, and took some getting used to! I'm not sure I could ever get used to driving around Beverly Hills in a Ferrari; but I don't mind doing that now and then as long as Wayne or Janet is doing the driving, and as long as they don't go too fast. And how could I not appreciate meeting some of the people we've met over the years through Wayne? It was just a huge thrill for me to go to a Hollywood dinner party with Wayne and end up at the same table as my favourite actor of all time, Kirk Douglas, who turned out to be a great person. I couldn't believe it. Wayne teased me about being such a big fan. I talked about that meeting for weeks afterwards!

Some of the happiest—and craziest—times during the '80s were those spent travelling with friends to see Wayne play. I remember the time Wayne was getting the Canadian Athlete of the Year Award. The ceremony was in Toronto, but the Oilers were playing in Chicago, and he had to rent a plane to fly to Toronto after the game to get there in time. He phoned me and said, "Why don't you guys just rent a plane in Toronto, fly to Chicago and bring me back?" We did: a four-seater with a nice pressurized cabin. Murray Angus, Charlie Henry and I went to Chicago, and I was able to get the pilot tickets for the game, too. We caught a ride to the arena on the team bus. It was the first time Murray had ever travelled on an NHL bus, and he didn't realize that the seating reflects a very important pecking order. We got on and Murray sat down, and I saw Wayne get this look on his face, which I was trying to pick up on. Wayne went over to Murray and said, "I'll let you know where to sit." Murray was sitting in the goalie's seat or something! There was a ritual to it all, and he had no idea.

Poor Murray, that was the first of two lessons he learned before the game. As we were standing outside the dressing room, the door opened and Murray went to walk in. Wayne came charging across the room and said, "You can't be in here, you can't be in here!" I looked at Murray in disbelief and said, "What were you doing in there? You go in when you're invited; you don't otherwise. That's sacred ground before a game. There is no fooling around."

My friends were amazed to see all the NHL tough guys, like Tie Domi and Marty McSorley, politely saying, "Hello, Mr. Gretzky." Really, so many players were like Jekyll and Hyde, on and off the ice. I always thought they were great guys, because they were always so nice and respectful to me.

WAYNE: My dad was always very popular with the other players. More than I think he realized. He wouldn't go in the locker room, ever, even though the fact was, he was welcome. He didn't have to wait for an invitation. For awhile there, he was the official unofficial photographer of the Canada Cup games. I mean, all kinds of people would be running around after the games, getting the players to pose for this shot or that one, but all the guys used to say, "If you want a photo, make sure you get into a picture by Walter Gretzky, because you'll get a copy for sure." That's just how conscientious and organized he was. He'd be on top of it. He'd make sure he'd get enough prints and send them out to every single person in the shot.

You never knew what was going to happen, going to those games. I remember one time, we were headed to a game in Detroit because Greg Stefan, a Brantford kid, was playing. His dad, Frank, was coming along with four other guys, and I was thinking, "How am I going to get six guys in one car in the wintertime, with big coats on—it could be uncomfortable." So Murray Angus said, "Well, I'll phone my friend Jack and see if I can borrow his limo." So we got this great big Cadillac limousine from Jack, a local businessman, and there we were, all leaning back, feeling like Mr. Big Shot. We got to Detroit, and Jessie Jackson had been speaking— that was when he was running for president. There were cops everywhere around the arena because he'd just left two hours earlier. We were driving around, unable to find a place to park. Traffic was gridlocked, hopeless. I said, "We're going to be late." Murray rolled down the window and asked a cop who was standing there, "Is there any place I can park?" The cop looked the limo over and then looked inside. I thought, "What the hell," and piped up, "I'm Walter Gretzky, Wayne's dad, and we're looking for parking." The cop said, "Oh hey, hang on!" He pulled back the barricade and said, "Follow me." He took us right to the arena. We got out of the car and followed him to the back door. This big tough Detroit policeman said, "You stick with me." He knocked on the door and shouted, "Open up, I've got Walter Gretzky here!" In we went, the back way. He said, "You want a couple of programs? Just a minute." He got them. My friends were delighted, and I said to them, "You know, I never, ever do that. But I think I'm going to continue!" It was true, I never did that sort of thing. Ever. I'd stand in line for tickets, and my friends would laugh and say, "Wally, for God's sake, just go tell them who you are." But I couldn't bring myself to do it.

After the game, we chatted with Wayne and had a little visit. Then we all piled back into the car. We were on our way home and feeling good, sitting there in the big limousine! All of a sudden, chug, chug, chug, stop. We were halfway between Chatham and London, and we'd run out of gas. It was three in the morning, a freezing cold night in February. We were all standing around on the side of the road in dress shoes. The wind was blowing. We had to go to work the next day. Murray said, "Oh Wally, I'm sorry, I forgot to buy gas." We all looked at each other and started laughing. I said, "Right, Murray, you ran out of gas, you go get the gas." So there we all were, at the side of the 401, wondering whether anyone was going to stop on the highway in the middle of the night and look inside a black limousine. Murray said, "Well, let's put the hood up, to show that we're stuck."

A truck driver came along a couple of minutes later, pulled over and drove Murray to the nearest gas station. Then he turned around and drove him back. Murray told him that he was at the hockey game in Detroit with Walter Gretzky. And the driver was this American guy who loved hockey. So, we got the gas. We finally got home about a quarter to seven in the morning. Travelling to the games was always an adventure. We'd make all these plans, and they would just not happen that way!

CHARLIE HENRY: On many occasions, back before Wally was widely recognized, we'd get into a taxi, and I'd say to him, "Well, where are we going?" He'd say, "The hockey game." And I'd say, "What's this kid's name, who's playing again?" And right away, the cabbie would say, "Wayne Gretzky." And I would go, "Oh shit, do we have to watch this kid again? I don't think he can play!" Well, one time I said all this stuff and the guy just stopped the cab, and said, "Get out." He was furious. And of course, then I said, "It's just a joke. This is Wayne's dad!" Sometimes, Wally would con me into it. He'd say, "This kid, Gretzky, do you think he'll play a good game?" Right away, I'd jump in with insults: "He can't even skate. What are you talking about?" The cabbie would go, "You're damn right he can't play," and I'd say, "You wanna meet his dad?" We had more fun with that. Although Wally was more reserved in those days than he is now, he would get quite a kick out of that sort of thing.

I guess that's one of my contradictions: I'm a worrier who gets a kick out of foolishness and spur-of-the-moment things. I remember one time, Wayne went to Finland to play in the World Cup championship. It must have been the mid-'80s. He had invited Charlie Henry and I to come, but we didn't think we'd be able to because we were both working. Then, at the last minute, I decided, what the heck, we should just go. I thought I'd surprise

Charlie, who was a firefighter in Ottawa back then. He was sitting at the fire station that morning when I knocked on the back door. One of the young guys answered and went back and said to Charlie, "Someone wants to see you." Charlie said, "Who is it?" And the young firefighter said, "Walter Gretzky." Charlie didn't believe him. But it was me! I said, "Get in the damn cab, we're going over to see Wayne." He said, "Wally, I'm working!" And I just said, "Well, pick up the phone and make some arrangements."

So Charlie got some time off, called his wife, Nan, and told her we were going to Finland. We took off that day. We had no tickets. We were truly winging it. We flew from Ottawa International to Montreal. In Montreal, we looked up at the flight boards and scratched our heads. I mean, we had to be in Finland the next day. We were really cutting it close. We figured that if we went to Copenhagen, then Stockholm and then Helsinki, we had a shot.

We started the journey that afternoon, and we got to Helsinki the next day. The tournament was in Turku, another hour from Helsinki. So we got on another plane, a mail plane. It was tiny, and I am not the most comfortable flyer. All I could say to Charlie was, "This is gonna kill me." Anyway, we got there, jumped in a taxi and sped to the arena. We had taken four planes, it had taken us twenty-some hours, and we made it—we were just five minutes late.

It was the first game of the World Cup and Canada was playing. Again, we had no tickets. Wayne didn't know we were coming. We were stuck outside, all these Finnish policemen were milling around, and we couldn't communicate to anyone why it was they should let these two crazy Canadians with no tickets into the game. I'm a law-abiding person, and I thought, "We're done here. We tried our best, but we're not going to make it." But Charlie looked at me and said, "Wally, I didn't come all this way to miss the game. Why don't we make a run for it?"

I had no idea how we would pull that off. I said, "Okay, but don't get me in trouble."

Charlie's a bigger guy than me, and he meant business. "Wally, just hang on to my coat," he said. "When I tell you to go, go." So I'm hanging on to his coat, and we're walking around looking for a door to crash. We went by one door, and this big security guy turned his back for a moment. Charlie just ran in with me literally on his coattails, and the guard turned around and started screaming at us. As we were running down the hallway, I could hear all kinds of people yelling behind me, and I thought, "Oh, this was a mistake! What were we thinking?" I was sure we'd get nabbed and hauled away to jail. Then Charlie saw an opening going down to the ice, where he could see a net. We kept on running, me still clinging to his coat, and then he saw the blue line and said, "This is it!" We went right by another security guy and ran down the stairs. The security guys were catching up to us. It was dumb luck, but we ran right down to the Canadian bench. Charlie had picked the right opening by chance.

Paul Coffey turned around and looked like he couldn't believe what he was seeing. He said, "Hey, Wally!" and got up. Wayne was on the ice. Then security jumped all over us. The players, hearing all the noise, were looking around, wondering what was going on. Everybody was running, following us. The Canadian players opened the door and tried to get us into the box with them. Finally, Alan Eagleson came over and managed to explain who we were to the security people.

By then, the game had stopped. Wayne, completely shocked, came up and said, "What are you guys doing here?" And we said, "It's okay. Don't worry about us." And Wayne and Paul started killing themselves laughing. We stopped the game!

Finally we were ushered upstairs to a VIP box, and we watched the game in great comfort, feeling immensely relieved that we hadn't been arrested. Afterwards, we didn't know how we were going to get back home. We went into the dressing room—by this time we were just part of the gang, Charlie and me—and the players were beside themselves laughing again. I said to Wayne, "Well, how are we going to get back to Helsinki?" He said, "You can't go back with us. The bus is packed. There's no room." He called over some organizers, and they put us on the VIP bus. I couldn't believe it. We were in these big roomy seats, and we got cigars, champagne and a waitress to serve us. There were about fifteen of us—Charlie, me, and a bunch of NHL owners—in a bus with twenty seats. Wayne was staring over at us in disbelief from the players' bus, where he and everyone were all crammed in. We just couldn't believe our luck. So we were sitting down with our cigars, and Charlie said to me, "We really pulled this one off." I just shook my head and said "I don't know how we did it!"

Charlie would get me into the strangest situations. I remember during the 1998 Olympics in Nagano, Japan, we ended up on the bullet train. I was in a good mood, just fooling around, and I started waltzing around the car, singing "When Irish Eyes Are Smiling." Charlie was egging me on, and he said, "Wally, why don't you take off your cap." So I did. There I was with my hat out, and, of all things, an elderly lady put some money in it! Charlie was just beside himself laughing. I felt terrible and kept trying to return the money to the kind Japanese lady, but she refused to take it back. Charlie never lets me hear the end of that one: Walter Gretzky, begging for money on the Nagano train.

Another time, Wayne called Charlie and said, "Would you take my dad to the races?" Before I knew it, we were on the Concorde, on our way to Paris to see one of the horses co-owned by Wayne and Bruce McNall compete in a big race. Bruce's people had booked us into this unbelievably expensive hotel, the Ritz Carlton, one of the most luxurious places in the world. Each of us had our own huge room. Charlie took one look, got his bag, came to my room and said, "Wally, let's get another place to stay. Wayne's spending way too much here." I had an even bigger room than he did! This is no lie: the bed was about ten feet wide. I felt as uncomfortable as Charlie did and got kind of mad about it. I called Bruce's office and got one of his financial people. I started chewing him out, saying, "Why are you spending Wayne's money like this? Charlie's not staying in his room, and I'm not staying in my room. Get us a hotel that makes more sense for us." And the guy said, "Don't worry, Bruce is taking care of the tab." I said, "Well, I don't care who's picking up the tab, we're not staying." The guy said, "It's too late now, Walter. It's eleven o'clock, and we can't make any changes." So we stayed there, but Charlie didn't go back to his room. There was more than enough space for the two of us in mine. The next morning we cancelled Charlie's room, but we couldn't persuade them to move us somewhere else. So reluctantly, we stayed there for three days.

Now this story is a classic. We were watching the race, and Wayne and Bruce's horse was running, and Bruce was back in L.A. One of his people was supposed to give him a description of the race over the phone, but she didn't know how to do it. Charlie and I were in our seats and heard her talking to Bruce, describing the race: "Well, Bruce, we're in first place. We're heading for the first post, and we're going pretty good. Everything is going fine." But Charlie and I noticed that a man sitting nearby was actually telling the woman what was going on and she was repeating it into the phone. It was one to the other to Bruce as the race was taking place. There was just one problem. I heard the woman telling Bruce that his horse was in first place. I leaned in and said to Charlie, "Are you looking at the same race as I am?" Finally, I turned to the lady and asked her the same question. She said, "Yes." I said, "Well, you're looking at the wrong horse. Our horse is sixteen, and he is in sixteenth place." The man says, "Oh my God." The lady said, "So now it's, uh, well, Bruce, I think we're falling a little behind." And when the race was over, that horse was last.

Afterwards, we went downtown, where there was supposed to be a celebration party, but no one was in a big mood to celebrate. Apparently, the day before the race, they had refused $8 or $9 million for that horse. So the victory party was really more of a wake. We were all eating steaks, and I couldn't help whispering to Charlie, "I wonder if this is the old nag itself."

After the party, everyone climbed into their limos to leave.

Charlie and I were sick of all the trappings and decided it was a nice night and we'd walk back to the hotel through the streets of Paris. Well, we got lost. We tried to hail a cab but no one would stop for us—I guess they don't pick up people off the street in Paris at night. We ended up flagging down a garbage truck and the driver kindly drove us back to the doors of the Ritz Carlton. Bet the doorman of that hotel had never seen guests arrive in a garbage truck before!

I've met a lot of celebrities over the years, and I'll tell you, one of the greatest was John Candy. I don't know why he and I hit it off so well, but we did. We'd just laugh and laugh. He was a fan of Wayne's, and I got to know him when he and Wayne co-owned the Toronto Argonauts for a time with Bruce McNall. I don't think I missed a single Argos game.

WAYNE: I remember we had just bought the Argos and we were sitting in the box watching the game, which the team lost. And after the game, my dad came out and said to me, "Did you really buy this team?" I said, "Yes, Dad," and he looked at me and said, "You need your head read!" I should have known my dad, of all people, would turn out to be right.

One time, Bruce McNall decided he was going to sign Rocket Ishmail to the team, and he said to my dad, "Walter, with Rocket Ishmail I'm going to do for Canadian football what Wayne did for hockey in the United States." I'll never forget, my dad just turned and looked at Bruce and said, "You're a damn fool. There's only one Wayne."

John Candy flew Butch and me to every Toronto away game in his private plane. He'd lay on a spread and we'd eat and laugh our way coast to coast. Charlie also had the chance to meet him when Wayne arranged for us to fly back to Toronto from a game in L.A. with John. Poor Charlie. John was a heavier smoker than I was, and between the two of us, we created a fog so thick in there you could hardly see. I was really sad when John died so young, and I miss him. I was still recovering from my stroke and missed his funeral. I also missed the highlight of his time owning the Argos. I had my stroke in October 1991 and that was the fall the Argos went on to win the Grey Cup.

I also once met Larry Hagman, when we appeared on a fishing show together. Old J.R.! This was after he'd rehabilitated himself. He'd had some bad alcohol problems, which he freely admitted. He'd even had a liver transplant since he'd done so much damage to his own. I found him very gracious, funny, down to earth and genuinely concerned about other people. That impressed me. We could talk about anything, tease each other. Maybe he felt he was making up for lost time, I don't know, but he has done his bit for charity, and I respect people who do that.

Wayne's brought home quite an interesting mix of people over the years. I'll never forget the time we ended up with KGB agents in our living room. This was when Wayne was playing in the Canada Cup tournament in Hamilton in the late '80s. That was some of the best hockey you'd ever see. Mario Lemieux and Wayne playing together—that was fantastic. One day, Wayne phoned up and said to his mother, "I'm bringing some people home for a barbecue." Next thing you knew, we were entertaining half a dozen

Russian hockey players, including the goaltender, Tretiak, and the coach, Tikanov, in our backyard. And sitting on our couch were two big, burly guys in suits, looking very uncomfortable. I invited Murray Angus over, and he asked me, "Who are they?" You should have seen the look on his face when I said, "KGB." In my house, in Brantford! It was pretty unbelievable. But the players were having a great time, and we were, too. Half of them didn't speak English, but they learned how to say "hamburger" soon enough.

Tretiak was kind of angry that these agents had to tag along. They were referred to as the interpreters, and they travelled with the team as security. Wayne managed to get the players past them and downstairs, one at a time, to have a cold beer without their coach or the KGB knowing. Tikanov was a gruff-looking guy, and I was scared that they'd get caught. But Wayne posted someone at the top of the stairs and took the players downstairs where the trophies were. They weren't supposed to drink at a tournament, strict orders. They couldn't have a beer, nothing. I suppose it was one time I didn't insist on being a stickler for rules! It was still pretty dicey with the Soviet Union back then. You really saw the differences between the teams after the game: all the Canadian guys would be coming out in their $3000 Armani suits, while the Russians were wearing zip-up track pants, carrying a little bag with their stuff in it and heading back to the hotel.

Wayne got to be great friends with Tretiak, and we once had dinner at his place in Russia. We've also visited places like the Berlin Wall, the day before it came down. It was quite a creepy feeling, going through Checkpoint Charlie, seeing all the soldiers patrolling with their guns, and looking at the places where people

Mary and Tony Gretzky, with Walter, on their cucumber farm near Canning, Ontario

Walter's first school picture, class of 1943. He's in the middle of the front row.

Walter, centre right, playing Junior B hockey with the Woodstock Warriors. He had NHL dreams and skills, but he was too small. Below, second from left in the front row, with the Princeton Panthers. Walter's friend Warren MacGregor is in the middle row, second from left.

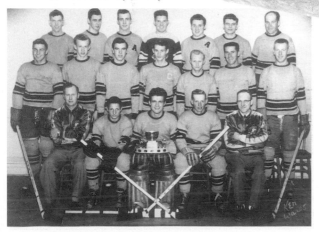

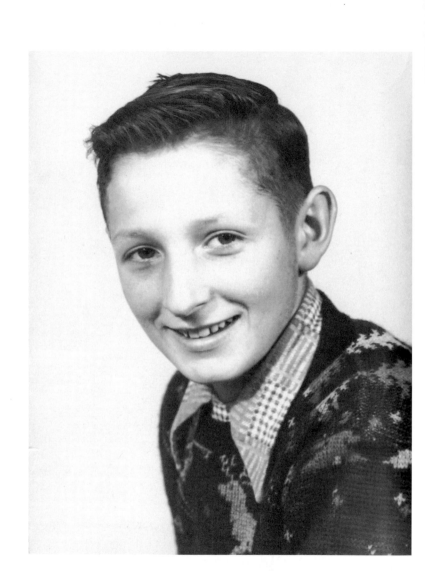

"Walter's kind of like Wayne, you know," says Walter's brother, Albert Gretzky. "He was smart, he had talent, all the girls were after him…"

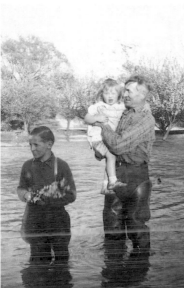

Walter, at left, with his father, who is holding Ellen, the year the Nith River flooded the farm

"I loved fishing. I'd go in the morning and wouldn't come back until late at night."

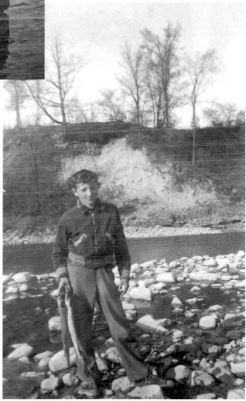

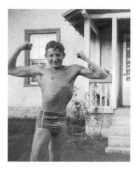

Hamming it up in front of the farmhouse

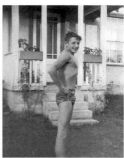

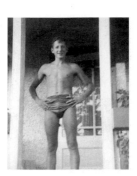

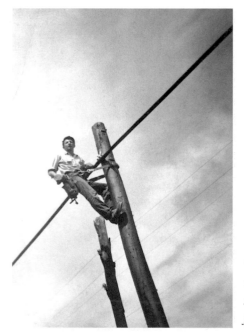

*Walter got on at Bell
Canada right out of high
school and worked there
for thirty-four years.*

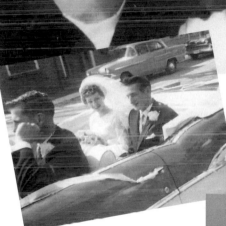

Walter met Phyllis at a wiener roast at the farm. She'd come with another boy but he didn't let that stop him. Left, leaving the church in 1960.

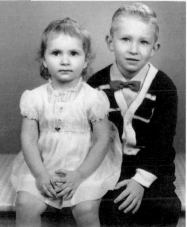

Kim and Wayne

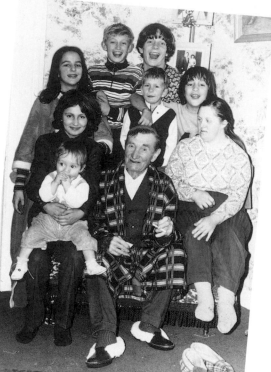

"Tato" with Ellen, to his left. Clockwise from left, grandkids Glen, Kim, Donna, Wayne, Kenny, Danny and Keith.

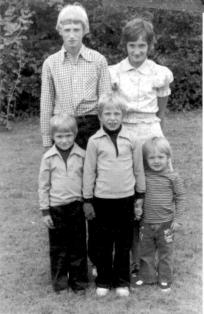

Clockwise from top right, Kim, Brent, Keith, Glen and Wayne

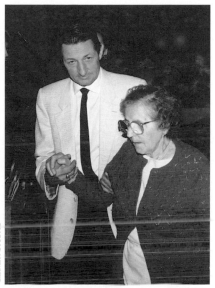

Walter with his mother just before she died; below, with Phyllis, delivering Wayne to the altar at his wedding to Janet in 1988.

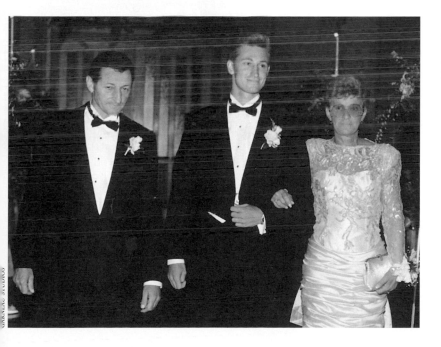

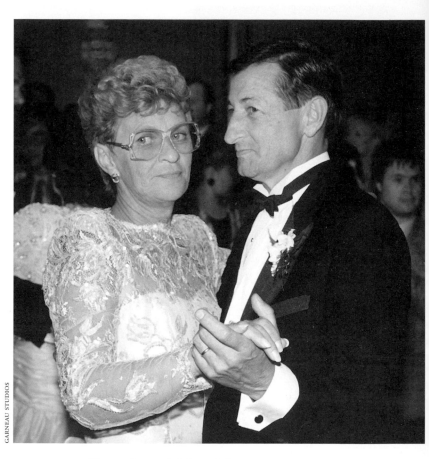

The mother and father of the groom

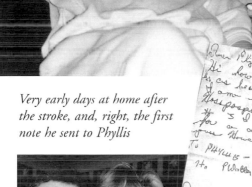

Very early days at home after the stroke, and, right, the first note he sent to Phyllis

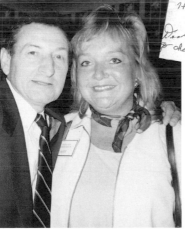

With Laurie Ham, the family friend who rushed him to the hospital

WALLY'S RETRIEVAL WARM UP   FRI. FEB 18, 1994

1 — WHAT IS YOUR NAME?
2 — WHAT IS YOUR WIFE'S NAME?
3 — ADDRESS?
4 — WHAT ARE YOUR KIDS NAMES? ✓
5 — WHAT DO YOU TAKE IN YOUR TEA? ✓
6 — WHO COMES ~~OVER~~ FOR COFFEE EVERY AM.? ✓
7 — WHO DO WE WORKOUT WITH ON MON, WED, FRI? ✓
8 — IT IS NOT PING PONG IT IS? ✓
9 — WHERE DOES WAYNE LIVE? ✓
10 — WHERE DOES KIM WORK? ✓
11 — WHO IS YOUR BARBER? ✗
12 — WHERE IS WAYNE'S RESTAURANT? ✓
13 — WHERE DID YOU WORK FOR 34 YEARS? ✗
14 — NAME TWO GUYS YOU WORKED WITH. ✓
15 — WHERE DID YOU PLAY JUNIOR HOCKEY? ✓
16 — WHERE IS THE FARM? ✓
17 — HOW MANY ACRES? ✓
18 — WHAT KINDS OF FISH IN THE NITH? ✓
19 — WHAT'S KIM'S DOG'S NAME? ✓
20 — WHAT COLOUR IS HE? ✓
21 — WHAT ARE YOUR BROTHER'S + SISTER'S NAMES? ✓
22 — WHERE DOES ELLEN GO EVERYDAY? ✓
23 — WHAT ARE 3 THINGS YOU PLANT IN THE GARDEN? ✓
24 — WHAT IS THE CLOSEST TOWN TO CANNING? ✓
25 — WHAT CAUSED THE DENT IN THE BRIDGE? ✓

Careful planning and mental exercises (above) designed to bring Walter back to where he could function independently

WALTER'S DAILY SCHEDULE

0930 – 1000	WAKE UP / PILLS / COFFEE
1000 – 1030	ADL (MORNING ROUTINE)
1030 – 1100	TO FARM (GET PAPER)
1100 – 1130	READ PAPER
1130 – 1200	EXERCISE (RIDE BIKE, ETC)
1200 – 1230	LUNCH
1230 – 1300	REST
1300 – 1330	REST
1330 – 1400	ATTENTION EXERCISES
1400 – 1430	TEA BREAK
1430 – 1500	WALK
1500 – 1530	WORK OF SOME SORT
1530 – 1600	
1600 – 1630	FINISH WRITING IN BOOK
1630 – 1700	DRIVE HOME FOR DINNER

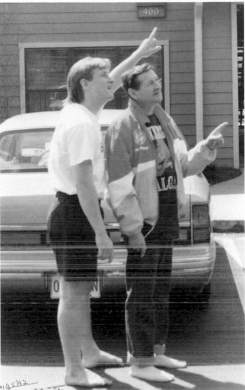

Walter with Ian Kohler, the therapist who became his son-in-law, outside Brent Gretzky's condo in Atlanta in 1993

The checklist Walter had to use to get through his morning routine in rehab

GOOD MORNING WALLY

DATE: Fri 8.5.92

DONE	INSTRUCTION (TICK WHEN DONE)	FOR STAFF USE
	1. PUT ON YOUR ROBE	Jnd
	2. PUT ON YOUR SLIPPERS	Jnd
✓	3. GO TO THE BATHROOM	Jnd
✓	4. USE THE TOILET	Jnd
✓	5. GO INTO THE SHOWER	Jnd
✓	6. TURN ON THE SHOWER	Jnd
✓	7. CLOSE THE ORANGE CURTAIN	Jnd
✓	8. PUT THIS LIST ON THE SHELF	Jnd
✓	9. UNDRESS AND PUT CLOTHES ON THE CHAIR.	Jnd
	10. STEP INTO THE SHOWER, AND USE THE CARD ON THE WALL	Jnd
✓	11. PUT ON ROBE AND SLIPPERS	IJP
✓	12. GO TO THE SINK	Jnd
✓	13. SHAVE (SUPPLIES BEHIND MIRROR)	Jnd
✓	14. BRUSH TEETH (SUPPLIES BEHIND MIRROR)	GJP
✓	15. COMB HAIR	Jnd
✓	16. GO TO YOUR BEDROOM	Jnd
✓	17. GET DRESSED	Jnd
✓	18. HANG UP ROBE	Jnd
✓	19. MAKE BED	
✓	20. GET GLASSES, BOOK, WALLET AND COMB	IND
✓	21. MEET STAFF IN DINING ROOM	IND
	HAND THIS IN TO STAFF LINDA	

HAVE A GREAT DAY WALLY !!!!

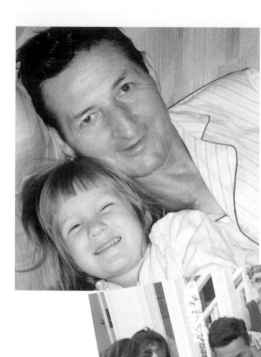

At home, cuddled up with Kayla, Keith's oldest child

At Ty's birthday party

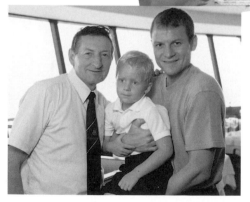

With Ian, and Walter's grandson Nathan in 2000

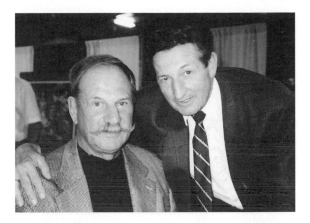

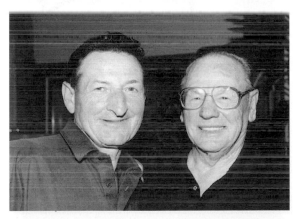

With hockey icons Eddie Shack, Johnny Bauer and Wayne Gretzky

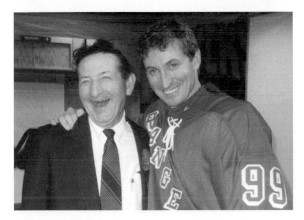

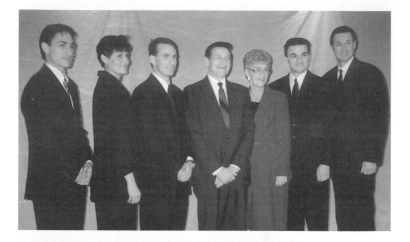

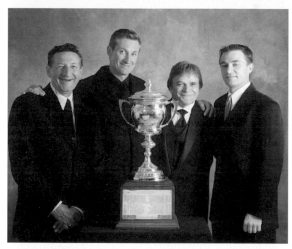

*One of the few
times in recent
years that the
whole family has
been together, at
Wayne's induction
into the Hockey
Hall of Fame.
From left, Brent,
Kim, Keith,
Walter, Phyllis,
Glen and Wayne.
Left, Walter,
Wayne, Butch
Steele and Glen,
celebrating the last
time Wayne won
the Lady Byng
Memorial Trophy
for most
gentlemanly player.*

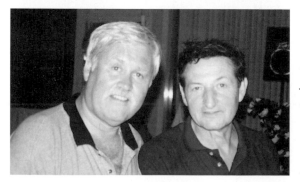

*With good friend
Ron Finucan*

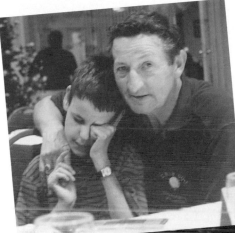

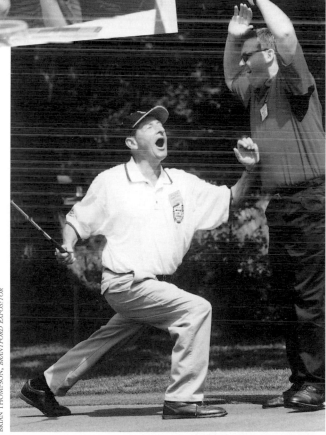

Walter and Daniel, left. And on the golf course, below: "The craziest swing known to mankind, but it works for me."

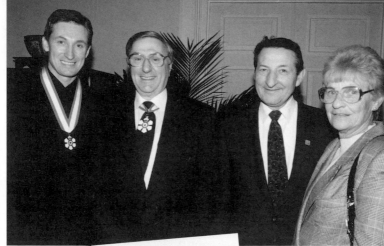

One of the Gretzky family's proudest moments was when Wayne was awarded the Order of Canada by then-Governor General Roméo LeBlanc.

Walter on Phyllis, his wife of forty-one years: "I joke about the fact that she's the boss, but it's true!"

had lost their lives trying to escape to the West. I wanted to get out of there as soon as I could. Another place that I'll never forget was Auschwitz. You see something like that and wonder how human beings can do such things to each other. It boggles my mind; it truly is almost impossible to comprehend.

I'd always wanted to go to Poland, to see the place my mother came from, and visit some of the old relatives. Again, it was Wayne who made that possible, and I travelled with Charlie and my other dear friend John Mowat. John had been a hockey scout for some years, and he had always been interested in baseball. He worked with Wayne as a pitching coach when Wayne was a kid. John and I had also co-owned a baseball team in Brantford together. He and his wife, Mary, were close friends of ours, and their kids knew our kids well, too. That trip to Poland is a memory I cherish, but it makes me very sad, too. In the middle of our trip, John had a fatal heart attack. He had been a healthy guy in his fifties who'd just had a clean bill of health from his doctor. We had no idea he had any heart problems. It was difficult to negotiate with the Polish authorities the transport of his remains back home. The red tape was unbelievable. It wasn't until Wayne called the Canadian embassy that we got any action. It was tragic that the trip ended that way, but the one thing that gives me comfort is that I know John had an incredible time. We visited an ancient church the day before he died, and I can still see John turning to me and saying, "Thank you, I'll always remember this." To this day, I keep a picture of the three of us on that trip on the desk in my den.

As I've said before, one of the things that makes me most proud of my kids is that they have all turned into people who want to give to others. Our family has been very involved over the years with the CNIB. That happened because of Wayne. He was about eighteen years old, waiting at the airport for his ride home to Brantford, and two boys who were coming up to attend the school here were also waiting. Wayne went over, and while he was talking to them, one of the boys interrupted him—both of these kids were totally visually impaired—and said, "I know who you are. You're Wayne Gretzky, aren't you?" At about one o'clock that night I just wanted to go to bed, because I had to get up and go to work in the morning, and Wayne was sitting at the kitchen table, so impressed that this young boy knew who he was by his voice. Not only did the boy know who Wayne was, he knew everything about him: where he played, some of the problems he'd already encountered, some of the records he'd held. And I remember Wayne sitting there at the table, saying, "There's got to be some way we can help kids like that. You know what we should do, Dad? We should have a little tennis tournament. I'll phone a few of my friends, and we'll have a tournament. We'll raise a few dollars for the CNIB. Well, eleven years, lots of tennis (and baseball) and $3 million later, that came to a stop, only because I had my aneurysm. Since then, we've started fundraising again through the Walter Gretzky CNIB Golf Tournament, which takes place here in Brantford every July. The money we raise goes to a scholarship fund that helps visually impaired students from across Canada with the costs of going to university. Our daughter Kim administers the fund, soliciting applications and arranging for a jury to decide on the winning candidates. In the first year we awarded five scholarships, and now we are up to fifteen.

Those early tennis tournaments and baseball games were wonderful and exciting. They were a great boost for the community, with many local people getting involved. We even did a pioneer re-enactment one year, complete with townsfolk dressed as soldiers, firing off cannons and guns. The funny thing was, I guess I'd forgotten to tell Wayne what was on the agenda. He arrived for the tournament and was a bit puzzled to see people dressed up as though they were from the nineteenth century. It was 110 degrees out in the sun, and some of the people in their military uniforms must have lost twenty pounds in sweat. Wayne apparently waved our good friend Brian Cooper over and asked, "What's my dad doing, trying to start a war?" I guess he forgot I'm a history buff. Muskets and bagpipes are right up my alley!

We had sports figures, soap opera stars, rock musicians, you name it, coming to the tournaments year after year: Glen Campbell; Brendan Shanahan; the Leafs; Colin Campbell; Scott Stevens—what a nice guy; Bruce Hood, the referee; Kirk Muller—nice guy, too; Jim Kelly from the Buffalo Bills, six-foot-five and such a nice man; Marty McSorley, who came every year; Brett Hull and Gordie Howe—they were the first guys to get on the field and the last off after signing autographs. Brett Hull signed autographs for two hours after the baseball game was over. Stood by the fence till every kid was satisfied. He even outdid Gordie Howe, and Gordie never turns down anybody.

WAYNE: Those tournaments were among the few charities around where 100 per cent of the assets went to the charity itself—in this case, the CNIB. My dad worked so hard to make sure of that. And he was so appreciative of the celebrities who would come and give their time and not ask for anything in return. Sometimes people did at least want their airfare and hotel paid for, and I had to say to him, "Dad, they are giving their time. You have to give them something." But he didn't understand that, given who these people were. So when people asked for nothing, he loved them and would go out of his way for them. People like David Foster and Alan Thicke just went all out every year, and he felt indebted to them for making that tournament such a success in the community.

One year, two young players came, one from the Kingston Frontenacs, and the other from the Kitchener Rangers—I think they won a contest to attend. So we were standing in the VIP tent with these two kids who were seventeen years old, Junior A players and just drafted. Their eyes were bugging out, they had plates of food they couldn't eat because they were surrounded by the greats. They weren't looking at the Hollywood stars, they were watching the hockey players! Murray Angus took Paul Coffey, Mark Messier and Marty McSorley, the biggest guys he could find, over and said to the kids, "You guys want to meet these guys?" Messier, built like granite, shook one kid's hand, and said "What position do you play?" The kid said, "Uh, defence." Messier said, "Oh. Left-handed?" "Uh, yeah." Messier said, "I've never had much luck against you left-handed guys. Watch yourself." Those kids were speechless.

Dave Semenko, a sweetheart of a guy who played with Wayne in Edmonton, used to come to the tournament. Those original Oilers have become legendary now. Some are still playing. But they came to our charity events. I could see that they loved Wayne and would do anything for him, and we all appreciated it.

Other Hollywood celebrities who came over the years: John Candy, Donna Mills from *Knots Landing*, Cheryl Tiegs, Alyssa Milano, Rob Lowe, Brian Patrick Clark from *General Hospital*, Bob Woods from *One Life to Live*—that's who my mum liked. He was one of the nicest guys. Rob Lowe was young and cocky then, but he was very nice and polite. Shannen Doherty from *Beverly Hills, 90210* was supposed to be an incredibly wild, partying kind of girl, but she stayed here in Brantford and was nothing but polite and generous with her time, just an absolutely charming girl. Teri Garr, Connie Sellecca, Alan Thicke and Jamie Farr came, too.

I'll never forget Mike Levine, the lead guitarist from Triumph. He and his wife arrived late. Levine had tattoos, long hair and sunglasses, and both of them were dressed like bikers. They looked so tough, I admit, I did a bit of a double-take, thinking, "Uh-oh, here comes trouble." But nothing could have been further from the truth. First, he apologized for being late and explained that he and his wife had had to attend a parents' meeting at their kids' school. He was so friendly, and for the whole weekend was very open and pleasant and mingled with the crowd, having a great time. It was one of those cases where appearances can fool you— I do know it's true that you shouldn't judge a book by its cover.

My priority with those tournaments was simply to make sure that we raised as much money as possible for the kids at the school.

That was it. I didn't want anything to be too complicated, and I wanted everyone to stay focused on that fundraising goal, which was tricky at times.

My other priority was to make sure that everyone had a good time. By everyone, I don't just mean the celebrities—though I wanted them to be well looked after—but also the local people, who paid their money to see the celebrities play tennis or baseball. There were always a lot of kids around, our own, too, and relatives. I wanted to make sure that they didn't get overlooked in all the excitement.

After the tournaments were over, we'd invite the celebrities out to the farm for some private downtime. We felt that was important, because they'd been "on" for so long, and we wanted them to be able to relax. Those were some of the nicest times of all. We'd have a barbecue, and everybody would be lounging around on the lawn out there. It was the biggest thrill of all to my mother, who got to meet her favourite soap stars. They were so nice to her. The ones who came were the ones who had a lot of respect for Wayne and would never have done anything to embarrass him or his family.

DANNY HOPPER, NEPHEW: As kids, we used to be invited up from North Carolina for those tournaments. Walter was very good at seeking out things that we could do. You'd seen these celebrities on TV, but this was a chance to go and put a live face, and flesh and bones to the person. To find out how normal a lot of them were! Peter Barton, who was on *The Young and the Restless*, we had a good time with him, he was very likeable. We got time to talk to a lot of the music stars, Platinum Blonde, and so on. After one of the tournaments, at the get-together at the farm, Eddie Murray, Paul Coffey, Wayne, Keith, Brent and myself were out in the yard playing a little touch football. Big Wally would be in the middle of it. He would take the time so that if you wanted to meet somebody, he would introduce you. He made you feel as much a part of it as he could. For a lot of the stars, my feeling was it was always a joy. When they came to the farm, people were just like anybody else. I wouldn't say all of them, but a lot of them would come. You could let your hair down. We'd have two or three grills going. It'd be great. It was an easy time. The public eye wasn't there, the TV camera, the newspaper reporter. I don't know how they kept them away, but I can remember that nobody ever imposed.

Wally would stretch himself as far as he could, getting the stars to come and realize, let's all be down-to-earth here, have a good time. He was more at ease there than at the tournament. He was a bundle of nerves during the tournament, then afterwards, he would be, phew, we got through this. And everyone would mellow down.

MURRAY ANGUS: Walter was the final say, the beginning, the end and the middle. We didn't want to bother Wayne with stuff because Wayne wasn't here. He was playing hockey. He was busy, as he should have been. Walter fell into this role of being in charge. The first year, he stood back and just let us do it. And it went off okay. And then the second year, it started to grow. Wally started to get more into it. And nobody but Wally would ask the questions that people needed to answer.

It was funny, because he could relate better to the normal amounts of money as opposed to the $150,000 or $200,000 that we would raise. We would go in, and I'd say, "Wally, I need you to sign this cheque for $78,000 to Talking Books at the CNIB, and I need you to sign this cheque for $52,000, and we've got to pay this $214 phone bill. And he'd be, "$214! Oh my God!" I mean, the big cheques, he'd just sign them, but the $214 phone bill got the biggest reaction.

He wouldn't let anybody get away with stuff. He took this seriously. And with him, the simplest, easiest way of doing something was always the best. "Don't complicate things," he'd say. "I've never complicated my life." I'd say, "Oh yeah, right. Wayne's career is not complicated?" And he'd say, "Oh, I don't know what happened there!"

Everything was simple with Wally. It was yes or no, it was either the truth or it wasn't. All these guys who were after Wayne's career back then, they all had briefcases and suits. They had companies and legal departments, and they would shake his hand, and then it wouldn't happen the way they said. But the thing about Wally, you couldn't pull the wool over his eyes.

Murray's right, I did want to keep things simple, and I didn't have patience with people who tried to complicate things or get greedy. The tournament became a corporate sponsorship. It was funny, because the local committee would meet the sponsors, and the sponsors would be a big, flashy presence, maybe pushing the committee around a little bit. I would go to the meeting, and suddenly, they'd behave. I'd say to them, "What you get out of this as a promotion, that's up to you. All I want to make sure of is that those kids get money at the end." After eleven years, the corporate guys wanted more. So we would have to put up bigger tents and do more promotion, and justifiably so, because the sponsors were putting up a lot of money. But they lost sight of the fact that all I wanted to do was make sure the blind kids got knapsacks and talking books, and if they couldn't afford to buy a machine to listen to a talking book, someone would give them one. Simple as that.

The '80s were certainly among the busiest and most exciting years of my life, and I can't disagree with anyone from that time who portrays me as a chain-smoking worrywart with headaches and ulcers. There were many happy events during those years, many of them to do with Wayne and all his amazing hockey achievements. Keith and Brent were launching their hockey careers, too. I travelled around the world and met some wonderful people. Wayne got married to Janet in a beautiful ceremony in Edmonton in 1988, with many of our extended family members present (Wayne made sure of that). And Paulina, our first granddaughter, was born.

There were some not-so-happy events too, as there are in any family. Perhaps the saddest for all of us was the death of my mother, on December 11, 1988, only a few days before Paulina came to us. I was pretty devastated. We'd been so close. She'd been ill with leukemia for some time, and at eighty-five, had lived a good, long life. She was such a strong and supportive force in our lives and had lived to see her grandkids accomplish a lot, and to be very proud. We did what we could in her last days to alleviate her worries about what would happen to Ellen. I was so relieved when Phyllis agreed to take her in to live with us, and grateful—it's a lot of hard work to deal with Ellen, and you have to be committed to do it day after day, year after year.

The day of my mother's funeral, we formed a convoy behind her for one last drive past the farmhouse. It was important to me that we do that, in honour of her memory, and all the time she had spent living there, raising all of us, giving us the best chance she knew how to in life. The place feels diminished without her presence, but I believe her spirit does live on there, and, of course, we will never forget her.

I've told you a few stories here, and some of my friends and family have stepped in to offer their memories, as well. I hope I've captured some of the flavour of what it was like during those years. But I must emphasize that I've had help re-constructing these events in my life. After what happened to me in 1991, my memories from about the late '70s to the middle of the '90s are virtually wiped out. That may seem hard to believe, but it's true. Everything you've read in this chapter, with the exception of the odd glimmer or small vivid recollection, is gone from my memory.

WAYNE: Back before his stroke, Dad was stressed to the point of no return. He lived on buttermilk to coat his stomach. His smoking was fierce. I'll never forget the Canada Cup championships from '87 to '91. It was great, because they were in Hamilton, so I could stay at home. But my dad was more intense about it than I was! He was so nervous, he could not even drive himself to the games. Someone else had to do it. I'd drive with him to try and get him to calm down.

It is no understatement to say that what was about to happen to me would change my life forever. I never could have predicted it, although in hindsight, given some of my habits and stress, the fact that I'd ended up in some sort of health crisis might not have been so hard to imagine. But at the time, nothing was signalling to me that the next phase of my life would unfold with any more difficulties or setbacks than it ever had. I just assumed, like most of us do until something happens to us, that I was in complete control of my future.

Well, as they say, the best-laid plans. . . . I couldn't have been more wrong.

chapter four

STROKE

I didn't have a lot to complain about in life, as the day began on October 13, 1991. I'd just had my fifty-third birthday and was five months into my retirement. I was getting into some new routines and looking forward to having more time for hobbies and outside interests, and more freedom to travel. I loved to visit my sons and spend time with my grandchildren. Wayne was living in L.A.; Keith was playing with the San Diego Gulls; Glen was selling real estate in Edmonton; and Brent was playing in Belleville for the Bulls. Kim was still living at the farm in Canning, working for the CNIB. We were all in the middle of planning a big fiftieth birthday celebration for Phyllis. I hope she's gotten over it, but thanks to me, the party never happened.

My world stopped that day in October. Just stopped.

I don't remember much of anything about the day, or the many days previous to it, or the many days of recovery after it. But with the help of people who do remember, I will reconstruct what happened. I am lucky that only part of those years are missing for me.

The farm was, and still is, one of the places in this world where I most like to spend my time, and with Kim there, I was able to go out pretty much whenever I wanted. It was a beautiful, sunny, autumn day, and I had decided to whitewash the old cellar, while Kim and her roommate, Laurie Ham, were at work. Though my mother had passed away three years earlier, her presence was still strongly felt at the farm, keeping us all in line.

The cellar was where my mother would put all her preserves, and there were still jars of her fruit and vegetables on the shelves. We continued to use it for storage, and I wanted to spruce it up. I was down there painting, when I was struck by the most terrible, violent headache. As I've said, I frequently suffered from headaches if I skipped a meal or hadn't slept, but this one had to have been the worst I'd ever experienced. I must have known that it was serious, and that I had to get out of there, because I dropped my paintbrush and made my way out of the cellar and upstairs to the kitchen. I've never finished that paint job.

One thing I am truly grateful for is the fact that Laurie Ham was at the farmhouse that day, because without her help, I am sure I wouldn't be here today. I knew Laurie well. She and Kim had been friends since their teens, and her dad operated a junior league hockey team in Brantford. It was unusual for her to be at home like that in the middle of the day. She had been away on a business trip and was going away again, and had only come home on the spur of the moment to re-pack her luggage. I find that quite uncanny.

> LAURIE HAM: There are some images in my mind from that day that are so vivid, and then a lot of it just swirls around. But I do have a technicolour memory of Walter coming into the kitchen from the basement, looking pale and shaky, and saying, "Laurie, I have a terrible headache. Get me a couple of Aspirins." I remember him sort of grabbing onto the counter-top as he said it. I got the Aspirins. He was dizzy and still holding onto the counter. You just knew it was bad, something more than a headache. I said almost immediately, "I think I better take you to the hospital."

I guess I didn't really put up much of an argument, which surprised Laurie, because normally I would have shrugged off going to the doctor, let alone a hospital emergency room, about a headache. Even though at the time she knew nothing about aneurysms or strokes, she had the presence of mind to get me to the hospital as quickly as possible.

Apparently, before we left, I wanted to change my pants! I'd been working in an old pair, and of course I wouldn't have wanted to go to the hospital looking sloppy. My mother's influence showing itself there for sure! But at that point, I got quite dizzy, and there was no way I could do anything but get into the car. I was still walking under my own steam, but getting weaker and more disoriented. Laurie wasted no time once we were in the car. The Willett Hospital in Paris is roughly a ten-minute drive from the farm, and she floored it. I wasn't saying a whole lot, but Laurie tells me I did warn her to slow down.

When we landed on the doorstep of the hospital, Laurie ran in, yelling, "I need help out here." They came out pretty quickly with a gurney and I was taken inside, and then I was sick to my stomach. It seemed we were there for a fair while. Although I was apparently conscious at that point, I don't recall any of it. Every time I hear the details, I feel bad that my family had to go through this experience.

Laurie called Phyllis and told her, "I don't want you to panic, but I'm at the hospital with Walter." Phyllis got hold of Kim, and they rushed to the hospital. The doctors told them that I was being taken to Hamilton General Hospital. They got me into an ambulance, and we headed to Hamilton in a convoy. I think at that point, the staff at the Paris hospital didn't want to say what they thought it was, but Dr. Hutton, the first physician to see me there, later said that he looked at me and knew it wasn't just a tension headache or a migraine, because of the fact that I couldn't lie down and was vomiting. He said that he just had a feeling it was an aneurysm.

By the time we got to Hamilton, I was unconscious and taken to intensive care. Kim and Phyllis were escorted into a little room set aside for the family, where they anxiously waited for any news of my condition. One of the best neurosurgeons around, Dr. Rocco de Villiers, was brought in to evaluate the situation. (I would learn later that Dr. de Villiers was in the midst of recovering from tragic events in his own life. The whole family marvels at the fact that Dr. de Villiers had the strength to look after someone in my situation at such a difficult time, and knows that without him I would not be around. We are very grateful for his courage and generosity.)

I think at that point, Phyllis and Kim still thought, "It's okay now. We're here, there's a specialist, this will be explained and taken care of." But then Dr. de Villiers said to Phyllis, "Can you call your boys? I think they better get here as quickly as they can."

PHYLLIS: On the day of the stroke, I was here at home, doing laundry. I was downstairs when the phone rang, and it was Laurie, saying she had taken Wally to the hospital in Paris. So I called Kim at the CNIB. She picked me up right away, and we went over there. We just thought it was one of his bad headaches, maybe brought on by the paint fumes down in that little cellar. He was sitting there in the emergency room, awake, and was able to tell me that his head was just pounding. They called an ambulance. Kim and I followed it to Hamilton. We didn't really know what was going on until Dr. de Villiers said it was bad, we should call in the family. Everyone was scattered all over the place, but they all got in. Then we just had to wait and hope for the best.

KIM: I had just come through the door from shopping for decorations for my mother's surprise fiftieth birthday party that my dad and I were planning when I heard the phone ring. It was my mum saying that Wally was at the hospital in Paris. I picked her up at her house and we drove there. On the way, Mum said that Wally had been painting in the cellar and that they would probably call at any moment and say he should take two pills and rest. We were both taking it lightly because he had never been sick in his life, and he had been fine when I spoke to him that morning.

Then as the emergency doors slid open, we could hear the sound of a man vomiting and Mum said, "That's your father!" He was sitting up in bed when we saw him. He looked over to my mom and said, "Phyllis, I'm so sick." But it still didn't kick in that there was a problem. All of a sudden, Dr. Hutton rushed in and said, "We're transporting Wally to Hamilton."

We got to Hamilton before the ambulance. Dad was still conscious and we followed him to his room at emergency where he stayed for about an hour, until a nurse said they were going to move him to ICU.

PHYLLIS: When I was told that Wally had to be moved to the ICU, I finally realized it was serious. I immediately called my sister Sandi, and she left work and came to the hospital right away. I knew she'd be able to help us understand what the doctors were saying, as she had had a brain tumour only a few years earlier.

While we were in the waiting room, Kim was on the phone speaking to Wayne. At that moment, Dr. de Villiers came into the room to give Kim and me the prognosis. Kim handed the phone over to the doctor so he could explain it directly to Wayne. With the three of us standing in a circle around the phone, we all came to understand at the same time the grave seriousness of the situation. The doctor handed the phone back to Kim—Wayne said he was on the way.

Kim and I went for a coffee to pass some of the time before the rest of the family arrived, and met Butch Steele, who had already heard the news on the radio and had come straight to the hospital. Later that evening, Sil and Mary Rizzetto came to lend their support.

KIM: I think they had done an angiogram by that point, and Dad was having blood vessel spasms, so they couldn't find the aneurysm. They couldn't operate until the spasms stopped, and this was really a risky period, when the worst could have happened.

BRENT: I was in Belleville. I had a game, and my coach called me into his office. I didn't know what was up. Then he shut the door, and I thought maybe I was traded or something! But he told me my dad was really sick. I left right then, went to Hamilton and met everyone at the hospital. I still didn't know really what had happened. We all rushed into the room, sat beside the bed, you know. We tried to talk to him. When you don't get any movement or anything from your father when he's lying there, that's pretty scary. It's something I wouldn't want anyone to go through. Definitely scary, and painful.

GLEN: I was living in Edmonton at the time. Around eight o'clock in the morning, I was going to work, and I was talking to Dad on my car phone. Everything was fine. He told me he was going out to the farm to paint the basement. We talked a lot on the phone like that. Casual stuff. A few hours later, Kim phoned, and she was crying. She said, "You've gotta get home. Dad's really sick." I tried to book a flight, and wouldn't you know, it's October in Edmonton and there was a major snowstorm that day. It was unbelievable. I was told, you are not going to get out of here today. Eventually, they re-opened the airport, and I was able to catch a flight to Toronto that got in around midnight. I went right to the hospital in Hamilton. And then we just hung around and waited. All we knew was that Dad was a pretty sick guy.

KIM: I think my dad's stroke was toughest on Glen. He always looked up to Wally, and though he left home when he was eighteen, he spoke to Dad almost every day. When he got to Hamilton from Edmonton, for a while he couldn't bring himself to enter the hospital because he was so emotionally distraught. Perhaps it was because he was the only family member who had to fly in on his own, and he had four hours to think of the worst scenario.

Following the stroke, Glen stayed at the house in

Brantford for three or four weeks (after everyone had left to go back to their "normal" lives) to make sure Wally and Mom were all right.

KEITH: I remember we didn't skate that day—we had some time off. The San Diego coach, Donny Waddell, and I went for a walk, and he said he wanted to talk to me about something else later on. Nothing to do with my dad. A couple of hours later, he called and said to come see him. I went and he said, "Your dad's sick. You need to call Mike Barnett [Wayne's agent]." I called, and they told me what happened. They were in L.A. So they flew to San Diego and picked me up. It was Wayne and Janet, their kids, me, my wife and my daughter Kayla. We flew into Hamilton. We went straight to the hospital. At that point, we didn't know what was going to happen to Dad. He looked so helpless.

WAYNE: I was at home in L.A., getting ready to lie down for a rest before a game. It was about 1:30 in the afternoon. I heard Janet running up the stairs to tell me that my sister was on the phone and that my dad was really sick. Kim said the doctors had told her and my mum he had only a 5 to 10 per cent chance of making it through the night, and we all had to get there. It must have been two or three in the morning when we finally got to the Hamilton airport. We were all pretty scared of what might happen. One of the people who met us there was a good friend of the family, Brian Cooper, and I asked him what was going on. He just said, "Wayne, I'm not a doctor, but from everything they're saying, it looks bad." Obviously, as with any family dealing with something like this, it's the unknown that makes everyone nervous. I don't think any of us knew what a brain aneurysm was, or what kind of chance my dad had for surviving what was happening to him. It was a long seventy-two hours. My mum was really the pillar of strength who pulled everyone through.

That was the first frightening period we all had to survive. By now, our extended family and friends also knew what had happened, and the local and national media were starting to run stories about my condition. Everyone was really getting prepared for the worst. Hard as it is for me to believe, it was big news, and many people were concerned about my condition. Telegrams literally poured in. Thoughts and good wishes came from the prime minister at the time, Brian Mulroney, from entire hockey teams around the continent, from school kids, and from ordinary people who didn't know us personally, but simply wanted the family to know they were praying for me. So many flowers were delivered, there wasn't room for them in the hospital, and Phyllis didn't want them going to the house, because no one was ever there—she and Kim pretty much moved into the hospital for the first weeks. So, they enlisted Phyllis's mother as the keeper of many of the arrangements. One was a massive plant from Magic Johnson, whom I'd met through Wayne in Los Angeles. It was so tall, they had trouble getting it in the door!

PHYLLIS: My mom and my sister Shelley were a big help. There was nothing they could do for Wally, but they were crucial in taking care of Ellen, handling all the telephone calls and making sure everything was fine at home. I'm not sure we ever thanked them enough for that.

Of course, I was unconscious and oblivious to all this. It's only now I can say how much I and my family appreciated it. Most of the expressions of concern were positive and helped my family feel supported at a very difficult time. There was just one unfortunate incident. a Toronto radio station actually announced that I had died. I don't know how this rumour got started, but as you can imagine, it infuriated those closest to me, because in the midst of worrying about me and trying to cope, they had to scramble to assure everyone that I was not dead! Our good friend Ron Finucan from the CNIB recalls that he was driving in his car, listening to the radio, when he heard the report and went into shock. He'd just seen me at the hospital, and although I was in rough shape, I was definitely still among the living! He and many others spent a few hours under the impression that they'd soon be at my funeral, before the confusion and distress were cleared up.

Meanwhile, there was nothing the doctors could do, because of spasming in the blood vessels in my brain. It was a Wednesday when it all began. They couldn't operate until the spasms stopped. On Saturday they did another angiogram, and within an hour of determining that the spasms had ceased, they did the surgery, which took five hours. Then they had to pretty much just wait and see how I would do. When Dr. de Villiers came out and spoke to my family, he said, up front, that I had had a brush with death. He said they actually found scar tissue, and that it was possible I'd had a previous bleed in my brain and didn't know it.

The kind of stroke I had is called a subarachnoid hemorrhage, which means there's bleeding on the surface of the brain, between the brain and the skull. This kind of hemorrhage is usually caused by an aneurysm, which is a weak spot on a blood vessel—probably something you are born with—and when it breaks, it causes a hemorrhage, and that in turn injures brain cells. Of course, that was only the beginning of my stroke-related problems. Along with the surgery done on me to repair the burst blood vessel, which, in the end, saved my life, I also had to have a permanent shunt inserted to drain fluid from my brain. You can see the tube under the skin on my neck, but it doesn't bother me.

When I finally did wake up in the ICU after all the surgery, surrounded by my family, I was utterly, profoundly disoriented—"completely out of it," as Glen would say. It must have been a difficult sight for my loved ones. I was hooked up to a tangle of tubes and machines. My hands were bound up in so much gauze it looked like I was wearing boxing gloves. My arms were tied down so that I wouldn't grab at the staples on the shaven side of my head. The doctors weren't even sure I'd ever open my eyes. (I finally did, of course, and I sometimes wear glasses as I did before, but one of my eyes will droop a bit when I am tired.) I'm sure everyone was anxiously waiting for me to say something, anything, and hoping that whatever it was made sense.

The first thing I did was speak Ukrainian to Phyllis, and Phyllis doesn't speak Ukrainian. Fortunately, my brother Albert understood that I was mumbling about feeding the chickens, and knew that I was recalling my very early life. I guess that was better than nothing, but apart from that, I couldn't remember a lot. I was extremely agitated. I'd say something in Ukrainian and be very frustrated when the person I was speaking to didn't understand.

After a short time, I did revert to speaking English. I knew who most people were, vaguely, but my sense of time was completely shot. It gradually dawned on those around me that my memories were severely scrambled or gone altogether. I thought Brent, who was nineteen at the time, was still a baby. I recognized my granddaughter Paulina, but I didn't know her baby brother, Ty. He'd been born in the year before my stroke, and that period really seemed to have been wiped out of my memory bank, along with most of the decade before that. That's what my family had to absorb and accept in those very early days, along with the fact that not even the neurosurgeon could tell any of us just how much of my old self I'd get back. The only thing they knew was that whatever recovery I did have, it was going to take a long, long time. Years, as it turned out, of hard work, perseverance and the patience of saints.

After a week or so, Brent, Keith and Wayne had to get back to playing hockey, but they kept in touch, phoning and visiting in the months following, whenever they could. Glen stayed on a few more weeks, and Phyllis and Kim resigned themselves to making hospital visits a part of their lives. They were really heroic about it, I have to say. It was obvious that I needed twenty-four-hour care and couldn't go home in the shape I was in. At one point, Wayne even suggested that I be moved down to California, where he had been assured I could receive excellent private care, but Phyllis steadfastly said no to that. She felt instinctively that it would be best for my recovery if I was close to home.

Fortunately, there was a spot for me in a small, well-regarded rehabilitation facility for people with brain injuries of all kinds at the nearby Chedoke Hospital, of the Hamilton Health Sciences Corporation. It was suitable because for one thing, the building was separate from the main hospital, so they could protect our privacy. There was a lot of attention drawn to my situation, especially when people learned that Wayne was going to be visiting me on and off, and my family wanted to keep the visits and my recovery as confidential as possible. No one wanted reporters wandering onto the ward. Because there was so much media curiosity, the hospital issued a press release stating that I had been transferred from Hamilton General to Chedoke for rehabilitation. They were just as concerned as my family was about maintaining our privacy. All visitors were screened before they came. I was absolutely in no shape to meet members of the public or comment on what was happening to me.

So on November 17, 1991, I was released from the hospital and to the unit at Chedoke, which is secluded and designed to be somewhat home-like, so that people can practice routines they'll follow once they really do go back to their homes. There's the main hospital, and then across a short field, there was a building that stood alone, called the East Cottage. There were five people in the program at the time, and I was one of them. Whether I knew what was going on or not, moving from the Hamilton General to this new "home away from home" was the first step along the way to being able to function again in the outside world.

Back then, it really was a question of taking everything one day at a time, and it was not easy. Phyllis and Kim recall coming to see me during my first week at Chedoke. I was eating lunch, and I started crying. That, they would learn, was another side effect that stroke victims frequently experience: a complete lack of control over emotions. One minute I'd be laughing, and the next, sobbing. You never knew what might trigger one of these episodes. It made no sense, and certainly was not my normal manner of being. On this occasion, Phyllis said, "Wally, why are you crying?" I startled her and Kim by saying, "Because they're so mean in here." Of course, this upset them, and they started crying, too. They asked me, "How are they mean?" and I said, "They're so mean to Butch." Now Butch is a very good friend of mine who would regularly come to visit, and no one at the place was ever mean to him! So they could tell I wasn't thinking straight. And I was still having such a hard time remembering things: where I was, why I was there. There were language difficulties, too, that lingered after I made the switch from Ukrainian to English. They would ask me what I had for supper, and if I'd had French fries, I'd say cucumbers. I knew what the right word was, but I was having trouble saying it.

It was a hard time. Hard on everybody, because nobody knew how much better I would get. My friends and family were faithful in coming to visit and happy if they got any kind of response or recognition from me. It's strange for me to this day to stare at photographs of myself from that time. It's like looking at someone else. But there I am with all sorts of different people. Bobby Orr came, and even Gordie Howe and his wife came to see me when I was still on the hospital ward. Although I only know this because I've been told about it since then (and have the photos to prove it), I am very touched and grateful to so many people for caring so much and taking the trouble to visit. I know it might not have seemed like it at the time, but I'm sure it all made a difference to my recovery, as little by little, I latched on to glimmers of the familiar, and connected together all the parts of my past, bit by bit, to form a whole picture that once again made sense to me.

GLEN: That first Christmas after Wally's stroke, we weren't sure if Dad was going to make it home. As it turned out, he was able to come home for a few days. My mum was having a Christmas Eve party for family and friends and I thought it would be a good idea to dress up as Santa Claus to lighten the mood and add some Christmas spirit.

I went to the front door and rang the doorbell. Dad answered the door, looked at me, turned around and said, "Phyllis, it's Santa." I don't know who was more excited to see me, Wally or Ellen . . . At that point, everyone in the house didn't know whether to laugh or cry, because my dad actually thought I was Santa Claus.

So I sat on a chair, with Ellen on my left knee and my dad on my right knee, and told Ellen that Santa would bring her chocolates, and I told my dad that although it was a tall order, I would try to bring his memory back.

A silence came over the room. I looked over at my mum and saw tears rolling down her cheeks. It was at that moment that I wondered to myself if my dad would ever be the same.

You might be reading this and thinking it all sounds awful, and in lots of ways I guess it was. But I still count my blessings. I could have died. Instead, I lived, and I had phenomenal care. I consider myself incredibly lucky to have met up with one individual in particular, who would be instrumental in helping me to heal from my injury and getting me back on my feet again. His name is Ian Kohler, and he was one of the rehabilitation therapists in the Chedoke Acquired Brain Injury Program. He was just a kid; twenty-two years old, starting a new career and paired up with me on my journey back to myself. When I met him, I thought he was the spitting image of Greg Stefan, another Brantford kid who made it to the NHL and was playing with the Detroit Red Wings at the time. "Stef" was what we always called him, and "Stef" is what I called Ian, although at first he couldn't figure out what I was talking about. When Wayne first met Ian, he said to me, "I see what you mean," because he could see the resemblance, too. I've said it many times, but really, without Stef, I don't know if I would have made it.

IAN KOHLER: I was always a hockey fan, always a fan of Wayne Gretzky. Wally's a pretty recognizable person, and when I heard about his aneurysm that October, I was watching the papers every day for any word on whether his condition had improved. About a month earlier, I was at a Canada Cup game in Hamilton with my dad, and I happened to see Wally, and I remember pointing him out and saying, "Oh, there's Walter Gretzky." Little did I know I'd be meeting him soon, and what kind of impact he'd have on my life.

A big part of rehab with a person who's sustained a brain injury is having somebody work with them hands-on, someone they can have a rapport with, someone they trust. Because of the background I have in sports, they paired me up with Wally as his auxiliary therapist, which meant that his treatment program was developed by the clinical director and by the senior rehab therapist and I was part of their team. I was probably a bit in shock after learning that I'd be working with him. A bit scared, excited, but nervous. We get some pretty challenging people who've received brain injuries. We have behavioural therapists and psychologists, and a high staffing level. It's really one-on-one. It has to be, for the treatment to be effective.

I remember the first day Wally came. He was transferred from Hamilton General, where he'd been in ICU and a stepped-down ward for one month after his surgery. Usually, once you're ready for rehab, you're no longer a medical risk, you don't need a team of doctors and nurses close by. When he got to that point, he was transferred to our program. He had a lot of rehab needs, but medically speaking, he was stable.

My first meeting with him was when I came in to work an evening shift the day he was admitted. They had a car parked across the entranceway of the East Cottage, with security guards, and I had to show them my hospital ID to get in and go to work! They screened everybody, and all the curtains were drawn, because we were prepared for the worst in terms of invasions from curiosity seekers and the press. Nothing ever happened, though. We just wanted to protect the Gretzky family's privacy and prevent the public from seeing Walter in that state. The first time I saw him he was playing pool, but somebody had to stand beside him or he'd fall over. Actually, he wasn't doing badly at the game, considering everything he had been through! The side of his head was shaved and you could see the big incision from the surgery.

Ian had had an opportunity to read my records and get some information on what had happened to me, but he really didn't know what to expect. I was unsteady on my feet, so I needed somebody to help me walk at all times. I had a really vacant look on my face—I can see that now myself, looking at those early photos. I was completely unaware of my surroundings, still pretty much in a fog. I was on a lot of medication, which contributed to that. I had no idea that I was at this place to get better. In terms of how bad off I was in relation to what they normally see, Ian says I was at the lower end of the scale of functioning. I was conscious but disoriented to time and place, confused and agitated. Communication was very difficult. I wasn't in a teachable state yet, but I had a lot to learn, or re-learn. I had a very fresh injury—from the perspective of a brain aneurysm, one month is still very recent—so Ian's goal initially was just to keep me safe, and the less stimulated I was, the better. If a person in this condition is in an atmosphere with a lot of noise and commotion, he or she becomes overstimulated. So it's best just to keep things low-key, and provide a quiet environment with a lot of assistance and reassurance. And that's what they did. Apparently, I wandered around that place for hours. Ian and the other staff would be with me while I tried to figure out where I was. I was saying a lot of things that didn't make sense. Mumbling a lot. All they could do at the time was make sure I didn't fall, and keep on reassuring me.

As time went on and I got a bit less confused, they needed to build some structure into my day. They knew I wasn't retaining any information. I wasn't able to remember from moment to moment and even second to second. Ian could say, "Wally, you're at Chedoke Hospital. You've had a stroke," and even if I responded, it wouldn't register. But by this point, I knew who I was, and I knew who my family was.

> IAN: What was so interesting was—we see a lot of people like this, and Wally went the same way—deep-seated memory is often there. Your ability to conduct yourself in a social situation, for instance. I can remember, he could be saying a bunch of things that didn't make sense, just be very, very confused, and then you would introduce him to somebody new, and he knew enough to shake their hand and say, "Nice to meet you." We call them "over-learned" things, behaviour that never seems to leave you. Conditioned stuff. I can remember him reaching out his hand and greeting someone, and I'd think, "Wow, you know, he hasn't lost that."

Well, it's nice to know I hung on to a few social graces through all of this, but Ian tells me that the thing that made me so challenging early on was that I was in a constant state of panic. I had this internally driven anxiety and restlessness. The intensity and duration of it was a bit unusual, he says, but you do often see it with stroke victims. The other thing about somebody who's at that stage, is that they always feel a need to be somewhere else. You're never content with where you are, because you are so confused and uncomfortable in your own skin.

As I got physically stronger, I just became more of a challenge, because I was literally moving around in a panic, looking for my family, even when the staff told me they weren't there. I constantly worried about my sister Ellen. I'd think she was in trouble. I continued to think that Brent was a baby. I could be talking to someone when something would suddenly pop into my mind, and I'd say, "The baby's missing," and run out of the room, looking for him.

It didn't matter where Ian put me, I wanted to be somewhere else. They would take me for a walk around the area outside, usually with two staff, because otherwise I would bolt. I would try to run away, and they would have to physically escort me back. They would put hockey on the TV for me, but that didn't seem to help at all. Obviously, it was difficult for my family to know what to do when they came to visit. It wasn't exactly peaceful. They could only do their best to restrain me from leaving the premises, and keep reassuring and orienting me. Ian tells me that sometimes I even tried to bribe him to let me out—"C'mon kid," I'd say, "how much would it take?"

I remember absolutely nothing of this. This was very early on. They had alarms on all the doors, because if they took their eyes off me, I was at the doors trying to go. They'd ask, "Wally, where are you going?" and I'd say, "I'm going home." But obviously I had no ability to plan any kind of actual escape. I would walk out in my T-shirt in the wintertime—that's how injured I was. When Charlie Henry was visiting one time, he thought I'd just gone to the bathroom when I'd actually left the building. He felt terrible about it and joined the staff when they went looking for me. It wasn't too long before they found me. I'd taken off across the field and managed to get quite a distance away, running in the opposite direction from home. I guess in my mind, I was being kept somewhere against my will. My family needed me, and I was determined to get back to them.

What was happening all this time, though, even if it didn't seem like it, was that my brain was spontaneously healing. Dead brain tissue doesn't come back, but over time the brain will try to compensate for areas that aren't functioning properly. With me, it took *so* long. A little, tiny bit every day. Two steps forward, one step back. The therapists would think they were getting somewhere with me, and the next day would be a disaster. I'd be at a point where I could manage to get myself out of bed and dressed, but then I'd be so disoriented and afraid, I'd run outside into the cold again at the first opportunity. And then the next day, I'd inch along a little bit further, and the next day, fall back again. I didn't have any physical deficits, but because of my cognitive impairments, I couldn't think to do things. And because I was in panic mode, I was more interested in finding Ellen or baby Brent than in having a shower or brushing my teeth.

I needed a lot of assistance to even care for myself. The hospital would collect data on how independent I was becoming. Probably the first sign of real progress was when I could shower, dress and undress myself. The fact that I was calm enough to even participate in basic grooming was an improvement. Gradually, over a period of months, I became more independent. I got to the point where they could give me a checklist—as is common with people who've had a stroke, I couldn't sequence even the most ordinary tasks. Generally, we all get up in the morning and know what our routine is. But at that time, I needed the whole shower sequence broken down into steps. I would look at my list and read "Take off your shirt." I had a pen and I would make a little check mark. I needed those cues. Ian would be right beside me, walking me through the steps and prompting me if necessary. The list instructed me on what to do, in sequence: "Put on your robe. Put on your slippers. Go to the bathroom. Use the toilet." I carried that list and a pencil with me, and I would check off each step.

In the beginning, for about a month, I didn't even know my way to my room in the unit. So, when I started to know where the kitchen was in relation to my room, that was another sign of progress. They got me to the point where I would wake up to an alarm. Ian or another therapist would enter the room and say, "Good morning, Wally. Here's your checklist for the day." They had a camera in my room, and they would watch me from the workstation. I would pick out my own clothing with the use of my checklist. I would independently walk to the shower room and take a shower and dress, and the last thing on my list was "Go to the kitchen for breakfast." Ian remembers the first day I did the whole thing by myself and they all stood in the workstation saying, "Yes, Wally, way to go!" Then it got to the point where I'd get a little smirk on my face when I'd finished my checklist, and I'd go to the kitchen and say, "Good morning." The therapists would all be so excited.

People are often angry and aggressive after a brain injury, but I was more confused and disoriented. I didn't have the ability to plan any aggression, but because I was in my own world, if you were blocking my exit, I might try to push you out of the way. I did that a couple of times. Ian would patiently say, "Wally, you're in the hospital. You had an aneurysm. You're in Hamilton," and I could get quite argumentative. I would say, "What the hell are you talking about?" I thought I was on the farm in Canning, and then the next minute I thought I was in Brantford. And then I'd say, "Ellen's drowning in the river," and Ian would say, "Ellen is not drowning in the river. She's at home with Phyllis." I'd be upset and say, "Don't tell me she's at home with Phyllis; I saw her, she's in the river!"

I was difficult to redirect at those times, because I was so passionate about whatever I was believing. Ian would try to maintain a calm demeanour and tell me, straight up, "This is the situation: you're in the hospital. Ellen's fine. Brent is playing hockey in Atlanta." But I couldn't absorb that. Saying that my baby Brent was playing hockey in Atlanta was like talking Chinese to me.

My days at the hospital were very structured, and I was not always happy about that. Ironically, after years of coaching my kids on how to succeed and persevere, I wasn't too interested, at that point, in having other people tell me what was best for me to do. But it was important in the recovery process to maintain the same routine, so that was one of the therapists' goals. They had me get up at the exact same time every morning, shower and have breakfast on schedule. The more I improved, the more they got me to do. Eventually, they got me to prepare my own break-fast. Even making a cup of tea was challenging at first because of my poor attention span, and because the sequencing of a task like that was overwhelming.

> IAN: My job was to work myself out of a job, because in this situation, as his therapist, I was his surrogate brain, his mental walking stick, which he needed until his brain healed and he got his mental strength back. I have to admit that working with Wally day after day at that stage was physically exhaust-ing and emotionally draining. I used to go home and have nightmares, he had me so wound up! You can place someone in what you think is a calm, pleasant atmosphere, but even that doesn't help. To this day, I would say that he was proba-bly the most challenging client I've ever worked with.

It was my high energy and constant panic that made me such a handful. Ian had to expend so much of his own energy when work-ing with me. There was never any downtime. Getting me to rest . . . I would not rest! And rest is important after an aneurysm. I would almost be crying because I couldn't settle. Ian would be sit-ting on my bed with his hands on my legs, saying, "Wally, you need to rest." And I'd be in tears, saying, "I gotta go, I gotta go."

I cried a lot. I got only very broken sleep. I would sleep an hour, just from exhaustion, and then I'd wake up. They tried to use the least amount of medication possible, because they didn't want to cloud my cognition any more than it was already. I would have been more heavily medicated if I hadn't been in a rehab facility. Initially, I would have only a couple of hours sleep at a time. I'd wake up and wander. Ian would be working the night shift, sitting and drinking decaffeinated tea and eating biscuits with me at three in the morning.

Ian, or whoever was working, would sit in the workstation and watch me on the monitor. If I stood and looked disturbed, they'd come in and do their best to get me back to bed. But half the time, I'd go to the kitchen and have some tea. I was always a little calmer in the middle of the night. I was still confused, but not in panic mode so much—probably because I was tired, plus the fact that it was quieter at night. But usually my sleep wasn't great, and one of the goals was to get me to have a good night's sleep.

We also did orientation exercises under the direction of a psychometrist, John Sullivan. Ian and I would sit together at a desk, and I would answer questions: What's the month? What's the day? How old are you? They would ask a lot of questions that they knew I had the answers to, to keep me interested—I liked to get them right!—and then they would ask me questions that I'd find more difficult: What is the date today? Where are you? What happened to you? And we went through probably thousands of trials, thousands. Because, like I said, as my brain recovered, I could retain more. It was just a matter of doing as much mental drill work as I could to get my brain literally back in shape.

I was also on a physical exercise program. They used to take me to the basement where they had exercise bikes and treadmills. The biggest barrier to doing anything wasn't my medication, it was my attitude! Getting me on the exercise bike was a challenge for Ian, because I simply wasn't interested. I didn't have any insight into what was going on, so how could they make me understand that it would be good for me to get on an exercise bike? That was always the biggest barrier: my inability to retain the slightest interest in doing something physical.

There's not a lot of research indicating that paper and pencil exercises are helpful with somebody like me, but Ian did them anyway, and I think they helped. I had such a poor attention span. I wasn't retaining anything, because I wasn't really making an effort to hear what anyone was saying. So they did some attention-training exercises with me, exercises as simple as listening to numbers on a tape, which would normally be a boring thing for someone to do. But I'd sit there, listening to the tape and writing out the numbers for maybe five minutes at a time. That's what I would do for five minutes out of the eight hours Ian spent with me every day.

> IAN: As rehab specialists, we're told to separate ourselves emotionally but be compassionate. With Wally, because I worked with him every shift that I worked, he came to know me. I'd walk into the cottage, and he would say, "Stef, you're here!" as if he was just really glad to see me. Because I spent so much time with him, I think he started to trust me. He and I really formed a bond. I get attached to all the people that I work with, but my heart really went out to Wally. He tried so hard. He had such a will. And even when he was at his worst, he was always looking out for someone else. He noticed the other patients who were in even worse shape than he was, and he'd sort of take them under his wing. There was one lady in particular, who was always looking for extra food, and we were trying to monitor her diet.

Walter would sneak food to her, because she was always saying she was hungry. You know, he just had that gracious, caring quality. It always came through. A true gentleman. All the nurses fell in love with him! When he got mad at me, I never took it personally. I felt I couldn't do enough for him. I stayed later. I would call when I was off just to see how he was doing.

It's easy to lose hope, because the process of recovery after that kind of brain injury can be so long, but I never lost hope with Wally. He had moments when I thought, "Well, if he can do that, if he can be lucid for one minute out of twenty-four hours, that means there's room to grow." There were moments when he would just sit down for a second and cry, and say, "I just want to get better." For that second, he would clue in.

I have the vaguest memories of cluing in for those few seconds that Ian talks about. Every now and then, I get a flash, just a small image, from that time, of me, sitting there thinking, "I don't want to be here. Please let me leave." I remember faces. Ian has taken me back down there to visit, and I recognized the supervisor, Shirley Holtrop, and some other therapists who worked with me a lot. I believe I even remember the lady who was always hungry. But mostly it's a blur. All I know is that the one thing I wanted most was to go home and be with my family. That was my entire focus, and resenting and hating the separation was the underlying feeling in all my anxiety and panic. I felt I needed to protect my family and was being prevented from doing so, for reasons I simply could not grasp. But when I went home for visits, I wasn't happy there either, and wanted to be somewhere else.

They say that the role of the family of someone who has had a stroke is as important as the therapists', if not more important, and that makes complete sense. The day I arrived at the East Cottage, the staff had a meeting with Phyllis and Kim to learn as much about me as possible. No brain injury is the same, because all of us have different personalities —the key to successful rehabilitation is not only knowing the type of head injury but also the type of head! So, they needed a lot of information. They learned about my personality and routines. They wanted to know who I was before the injury so they'd have some sense of who I could be after I left formal rehabilitation. And they want to gear your recovery program to what your life is going to be like when you go home.

> IAN: The family is always a huge part of a person's recovery, because it's what the person has to hang on to. I haven't met a family more dedicated than the Gretzkys. Phyllis and Kim were there literally every day. All of them, when they could be. I remember the first time Wayne came to visit, quite early on, and I knew immediately he was a good guy. He was very friendly and down-to-earth, just talking with everyone. Of course, there was a lot of excitement beforehand amongst the staff when he'd visit, but he put people at ease. He was just there to see his dad, like any other visitor, and you could see he really cared about him and wanted to make sure he got the best treatment possible.

Obviously, Wayne was living far away, and actually all the boys were far away, so it wasn't possible for them to be there physically a lot of the time. But they called the unit constantly and asked Ian or whoever was there for an update. Wayne would call almost daily as he was driving to the practice rink in L.A. or driving home, and ask, "How's my dad?" Glen, Keith, Brent, they all called. Kim, because she lives here, visited just about every day. She would bring Tim Hortons coffee in for the staff every evening. Phyllis was there, as well. They came together quite often.

I always had a ton of visitors. Initially, when they came to the door, the staff would say, "Sorry, we have to clear it with the family before we can let anybody in." My dear friend Butch came to the door one night just shortly after I was admitted. He had a bag of Oreos, and he wanted to see me. Ian had to say, "Sorry, I can't let anybody in. The family needs to screen who can and can't come." In his heart he knew that this was my buddy, but he had to make sure, just in case. So he called Phyllis in Brantford, but couldn't get her, and then tried to get hold of Kim, but couldn't get her. He didn't know what to do. He went into my bedroom and there was a picture of Butch on the wall with me, holding a big fish! So he went back to the door and said, "Come on in." Butch was another one who was there every single night. Didn't matter if there was a snowstorm, he would drive down from Brantford to see me. Ian says he was visibly upset just at the sight of me. We were such good buddies. Other friends visited too: Eddie, Charlie Henry whenever he could get down from Ottawa, Ron Finucan. And everyone was pretty excited the day Bobby Orr came to see me!

I was in the rehab unit for about ten months. To prepare me for going home, they would take me to Brantford for four hours or to the farm. If Ian was working evenings, he would take me home to watch a hockey game on the dish, one of Wayne's games, with Butch and Eddie. Taking me home on passes was all for therapy purposes, to reintroduce me to my own life.

It makes sense, really, that the best place for a person to recover is home, if that's manageable, because everything's familiar. But I wasn't ready to go home until August, 1992, when I was finally discharged. Even then, I was still in bad shape. I needed to be reminded of things and continued to have periods of panic. I think, looking back, that I made most of my gains when I went home. I made gains at the hospital with basic things like grooming and making myself a cup of tea, but I still needed a lot of care, twenty-four-hour supervision.

My family could see that they were going to need continued help, if I was going to keep getting better. Don't forget, Phyllis already had her hands full taking care of Ellen. Wisely, she approached Ian at the hospital the day I was discharged, and asked if he would consider leaving to come and work privately with me. Luckily for us, he said yes!

> IAN: I loved Wally. It was killing me that he was going to leave. So I went with him, and for the next two and a half years, he was my main guy. It was my responsibility to take him to the next level of recovery. I was determined to help him get better.

It's sometimes hard for me to believe that all of this happened ten years ago. Everything is so different now. We've all gone through so much. But back on that August day when I was finally going home, I'm sure my family felt some relief, but also some anxiety about how we would all cope once we were under the same roof once again. We'd had tremendous support from so many good people through all of the trauma of my injury up to that point. But we would need more support for some time to come.

One of the things I asked Phyllis when I got out of the hospital was to take me to the cemetery to visit my father's grave. I'm not sure exactly why I wanted to go: partly to pay my respects, maybe to reflect on my own survival, I don't know. Of course she said yes, and we went there together. She had no idea what was coming, and neither did I. When I got there, I looked at my father's grave. I was prepared for that. But then I saw my mother's beside it. That sent me into shock. You see, I had lost the memory of her death, which had taken place only three years before my stroke, and that was right in the period when my memory loss is almost complete. Poor Phyllis didn't know what to do. I just wept. I was thrown right back into grief over my mother's death, as though it had happened the day before. In my impaired state, it might as well have.

WAYNE: My dad was so close to his mother, it was a devastating loss in the first place. Then, he had to go through that trauma all over again. It was all so hard, more on my mother and Kim than anyone else, since they were there every day. We would see minor improvements, but then he'd regress again. We were not sure for the longest time just where he'd end up mentally. But he was always a big fighter, with a tremendous passion for life and people. Basically, it's a miracle he survived at all. They say things happen for a reason, and maybe in his case, having the aneurysm helped add twenty years to his life, because it forced him to stop smoking and take better care of himself. But it was a long, hard process.

Yes, coming home from the hospital was a milestone for all of us, and a welcome one. But the incident in the graveyard signalled to everyone that our hard times were not yet behind us. As much as we'd struggled and survived in the previous ten months, we still had a long way to go.

chapter five

HOME AGAIN

I must have been happy and relieved to finally sleep in my own bed, after surviving the stroke and surgery and spending ten months in East Cottage. I don't remember, and maybe I just don't want to remember. Back then, I had no sense of the impact my stroke was having on my family and friends. People were very kind and did their best to help me, taking the load off Phyllis and Kim whenever they could. Our next-door neighbour Karen Redpath took me for regular walks around the neighbourhood. At least once or twice a week, Ron Finucan would take me out to dinner and a movie. (At home, I'd try to watch a movie on TV and I'd just fall asleep or wander away, but at the theatre at least I'd stay awake! My old friend Warren MacGregor would come by at Phyllis's request and talk to me, trying to get me to understand that like him, I was retired from Bell and no longer had to clock in with my repair truck! It was quite the community effort.

But it was rough on everyone, seeing me in that state. Bryan Wilson recalls driving me out to Port Dover for a day trip shortly after I got home. Bryan and I were great buddies, and once upon a time, we fished together regularly down at Long Point. He always used to tease me about my black socks and black dress shoes, which I'd even wear to go fishing. He was having as hard a time as anyone coping with "the new Wally."

Now on this little outing, I didn't know where I was. We took a ride down to Port Dover and had a hot dog, and he asked me questions, just trying to make conversation, but I couldn't answer. I just looked out the window, working myself into a panic. Then I started arguing with him. "Where am I?" I asked. And he said, "We were just at Dover, Wally." And I snapped back, "Well, I'm not supposed to be here. I'm supposed to be at work in half an hour." Bryan couldn't settle me down, and I got really mad at him. It seems I wanted to fight. Finally, Bryan had to take me home.

Phyllis and Kim did their best to accommodate me and my new needs. Living with someone as forgetful, moody and, at times, downright delusional as I was at the time was difficult, no two ways about it. The doctor and rehab people had done their best to prepare my family for what life would be like with me in the house, but still, it was a dramatic shift. They were there to orient me every step of the way, patiently correcting me whenever I clung to some misperception. They even did things like label the drawers and shelves in the kitchen, bathroom and bedroom so that I would know exactly where everything was, and where to put things back so that I could find them again. This was the long haul.

It was only when I got home that the reality of my situation started to sink in for me, and frankly, it was depressing. This, I'm told, is not uncommon after a stroke. When I was in the hospital, I was in a kind of safe cocoon that allowed me to stay out of touch with reality. In the beginning, a person with a brain injury absolutely needs that kind of quiet, stable environment to go through the first stages of healing and recovery. But when I got home, on some level I knew that here I was, in the house I'd left the day I had the aneurysm, and I was not the same person. There's a sense of loss with that, some actual grief, even if I could not articulate it, which probably added to my sense of disorientation and made me want to hang on to the past I could remember. For the longest time, even after I got home, I remained obsessed about a number of things and clung to several misguided notions. I couldn't get it straight that my mother had passed away. Kim recalls one awful instance when I somehow got the idea that my mother was lying inside a large hockey bag. I would not let go of this notion, until finally my poor daughter, in great frustration, actually opened up the bag to show me that all it contained was some old hockey gear. I frequently thought I had to rescue Ellen and Brent from some kind of danger, and I still could not accept that I was actually retired. I kept on thinking I was late for work, or that my Bell truck had been stolen. On top of this, I had trouble retaining the most basic information, moment to moment.

> KIM: I remember one night, he couldn't find his watch. Dad, Mum, Ian and I hunted the whole house for his watch. And after forty-five minutes, Dad leaned up against the wall and said, "You know what? I forget what the hell I'm looking for. What are we looking for?" Things like that happened all the time. It got to the point where my mum and I finally realized that even though it wasn't really funny, some of the things he did, you had to laugh or you'd cry. Because it was pretty much just my mum and me, day-to-day. The boys had all gone back to play hockey. This went on a long, long time.

Perhaps hardest for those around me to accept, was the fact that all the things that had once been my life's passions—hockey, fishing, photography, working on the garden or at other chores at the farm—were somehow gone. I just didn't have enough memory or motivation to involve myself in any of it. I'm sure my family truly wondered what on earth they were going to do with me now. All of my grief and confusion over the negative changes in my life caused me to be withdrawn, and very cranky whenever anyone tried to get me up and doing things. That worried everyone. All they could do was keep on correcting and encouraging me, and have faith that I would get better. Without that, it would have been pretty hopeless.

Probably one of the worst moments for them came when they realized that I no longer enjoyed watching hockey. For more than a decade, Eddie, Butch and I watched all of Wayne's games on TV.

Even if the game was one of the L.A. Kings games and started at 10:30 at night, Butch and Eddie would be at the door. We called Butch "the chip man" because he brought the chips, and Eddie was "the donut man" because he'd always show up with donuts. Now Wayne would be playing, and Butch and Eddie would put the game on, and I just wasn't interested. I'd tell them to lock up the house after the game was over, and I'd go to bed. I think everyone was in shock, because, of course, before the aneurysm, hockey was just everything to me. I know this was a terrible thing for my family and for Butch and Eddie to accept. I think it was especially hard on Wayne.

WAYNE: It was really difficult, because up to that time, any decision I ever made, my dad was always my first phone call. He had more common sense than anyone I knew. He was my sounding board, especially when it came to giving me advice about actually playing hockey, and I had a couple of tough years when I lost that. I remember feeling it in particular during the Stanley Cup semifinals in 1993. I wasn't playing well. We were in Toronto, down three games to two. Normally, my dad would always be there to hear what I had to say. On my day off, I would have been able to go home and get him to calm me down. He was as nervous as a mouse himself, but somehow he could make me feel less wound up about my playing. It's funny, because he was always honest. He could tell me I wasn't playing my best, but in a way that built me up. I remember feeling it during that time, just realizing that I couldn't go to him for that any more.

BRENT: I remember, we'd be at the house and he'd be asking for me. I'd be sitting right beside him and he'd say, "No, baby Brent," things like that. I was nineteen then. That was a scary feeling. He was kind of distant. He knew from people telling him who was coming to see him, but I don't think he really knew who I was in the beginning. I'd sit there, and he'd still have a blank look on his face when he was looking at me. That hurt when you left, too. But we just kept going, trying to get him to remember. Just had to keep repeating it until he finally got it.

Of course, we were fortunate to have Ian with us, day to day. I think I would have driven Phyllis and the kids crazy (I did anyway) if it were not for his hands-on help. He did everything in consultation with the doctors and therapists in the Acquired Brain Injury Program. I was still under Dr. Garner's care. Ian was reporting regularly to him throughout the time he worked with me. He was on the phone a lot, discussing things like medication and any obstacles he saw to getting me further along in my recovery. Dr. Garner helped Ian understand what was behind my cognitive difficulties, as did John Sullivan and other therapists. If he needed assistance or wanted to consult, he could set up appointments. He would take me down to the outpatient clinic at Chedoke about every four months. We met with John Sullivan to do formal cognitive retraining exercises. They were just a small portion of my day, but Ian made sure I did the exercises religiously. I copied out numbers and answered questions, in order to help me attend to information, to think about what I was hearing and remember it. It took a long time, but I do think this helped me.

IAN: Because of Wally's condition, we needed to find a quiet place where he could get some exercise that was out of the public eye. Eddie Ramer made arrangements for us to work out at the S.C. Johnson Wax employee gymnasium nearby. We went every Monday, Wednesday and Friday morning. Phyllis got some relief, and Wally had an opportunity to gain some strength and conditioning.

At first he resisted any form of exercise to the point of me having to physically pull him around the gym. Table tennis is a good sport for improving physical and mental reflexes, attention span and hand-eye coordination. I encouraged him to play and reluctantly he did. Playing basketball and ice skating were other activities for Wally, designed to encourage independent functioning.

I remember the first time Glen and I took him skating. It was a major family event, with Phyllis, Ellen and Kim looking on with hopeful anticipation. For a man known around the world for teaching the world's greatest hockey player how to skate and play hockey, he couldn't even stand on skates. He needed the help of Glen and myself just to get around the ice. As much as we were excited to take him skating for the first time, it really showed the family that he was very much a different man.

I may have been a reluctant and uncooperative participant at first, but Ian did what he could to establish some routines in my life and help me stick to them. He would show up at the house around nine every morning. Usually Butch would be there with coffee for everyone, and I would still be upstairs in bed. That was the worst part of the day. Poor Ian could not get me out of bed. I simply would not get up. I was very stubborn. It got to the point where they were considering whether or not I was becoming clinically depressed. I was never diagnosed with depression, but my withdrawal and lack of motivation, my desire to sleep all the time, in bed or on the couch, and my irritability certainly were classic symptoms. I was shutting out the world. I didn't have a great appetite, either. For the longest time, all I wanted to eat was Kraft Dinner, which was strange because normally I didn't mind eating it once in awhile but would never have wanted a steady diet of it. For some reason, I couldn't get enough of it after my stroke.

Ian was pretty creative in figuring out how to get me out of bed! He didn't want to physically pull me out, so he got the most annoying alarm clock he could find. My bed was at one end of the room, and he would sneak in there when I was asleep and set the alarm at the other end of the room. The damn thing would go off and I couldn't stand it! I would have slept already ten, eleven, twelve hours. It was definitely time for me to get up. I do have a flash of a memory: me, darting across the room, cursing, to shut the alarm off. Then Ian would get in between me and the bed. Quite an ingenious intervention! He'd say, "Sorry, Wally. Nope, you're not getting back in there. There's the door, we're going downstairs for breakfast." And I would get so angry with him! It never got physical, but I would be furious. Butch and Phyllis would be downstairs, listening to all this, and Ian would be trying to get me downstairs. Eventually I started to become conditioned to the alarm routine, and then I got sneaky myself. I would try to beat Ian to the blaring clock and back to the bed! I laugh when they tell me about that now. I can hardly believe I behaved that way.

I still had moments of panic. Ian tracked them. From the time I was in the hospital, my caregivers kept a record of what they called my "worry statements." Ian had a counter, and he would count every one of them. When I was in hospital, there were hundreds of them a day. A worry statement was defined as something I said about thinking Ellen was drowning or Brent was in trouble, something that wasn't based in reality. The therapists were using a behavioural model of treatment; when you're trying to change a person's behaviour, these are some of the techniques you use. In my case, the problem was all of these unrealistic beliefs were based on my damaged memory. When I went home, Ian continued to track them. It was a good indication that I was getting better and calming down when the number of worry statements went down.

Ian worked with me for two and a half years after I got home. From the beginning, he would take notes about our activities and my progress. He was a great record keeper. Here's one of his notes from July 31, 1993: "Wally woke in a good mood. No worries to report. We went to Port Dover and all went well. At 4:30, he was unable to recall most of the day, but did remember parts with the help of verbal cues . . ." And another: "Wally was very difficult to get out of bed this morning. Approximately ten minutes to get him downstairs." This was when Ian was having to dance with me to get me up. I like this one: "Good spirits. Two worries." So I went from a hundred worry statements an hour in the hospital to two all day long! This is why all those notes were useful; we could really see that slowly but surely, I was making progress.

Still, every time I went on about missing work, Ian would have to say, "Wally, you're retired." I even sometimes used to think I was still in school. My mind seemed to want to go back to the days when I was running track. "I gotta go to a race," I'd say, and I urgently believed it. All Ian could do was patiently reply, "Wally, you are fifty-five years old. You don't need to go to a race." But I'd insist, "I'm tellin' ya, I gotta meet the coach. We gotta race today." One day, I was going on about this damned race as we were driving through Paris. Would you believe there was a race going on? The Boston to Brantford Marathon (there's a little town called Boston nearby). Honest to God, Ian was in the midst of assuring me, "Wally, you're not in a race," as we were approaching Paris, and then there were all these marathon runners racing through town! Poor Ian could not believe his eyes. And of course, I started panicking even more when I saw all these people running, and Ian had to figure out how to explain that even though there was a race going on, I didn't have to be in it!

IAN: Those times were difficult for Wally. All eyes were on him in the community. I remember once we went into the Canadian Tire store. I don't know what we were there to buy, but he was fine, and then his whole mood changed. He went into panic mode. In his mind, someone had stolen his Bell truck. And I had the damnedest time getting him out of the store. He was even approaching people, asking if they'd seen it. He wanted to report his truck missing. He was convinced

that he was at Canadian Tire to do a job. He had gone into all
those stores when he worked for Bell. So, all of a sudden, he
thought he was working and had lost his truck and his tools.
It was quite a scene, everybody wondering what was going on.
I forget what lie I had to tell him to get him into my car. I just
had to get him out of there and get him home. I guess I said,
"Well, you know what? Let's just get in my car and we'll go
find your truck."

To give an example of how argumentative Walter could be,
I recall a time when he was disoriented to the point where he
thought he was still in high school. Following several frustrating attempts to make him realize that he was no longer a high-
school student, I put him in the car, took him to his former
high school where students were mingling outside and said to
him, "Walter, look at yourself. You're fifty-five years old. Do
you want to join them?"

I really had no consciousness at that time of what other people
might think about me. I didn't want to do anything. To try and
get me interested in life again, Ian used to bring me out to the
farm for hours and hours. At one time I would have been eager to
go there as often as I could, just to putter around in the garden,
prune trees, look after the grapes, cut the grass. After I got home
from East Cottage, Ian would take me out there, because he wanted to structure my day. He would get together with Phyllis and
Kim and try to picture what I'd be doing in retirement. How had
I been planning to spend my days? Everyone knows you can't reha-
bilitate somebody at a desk with a pencil and paper; you have to

put them in real-life situations. Ian was just hoping that, eventually, I'd recover some of my enthusiasm for working around the farm.

For awhile, he had me out there every day. He'd say, "Okay Wally, we have to cut the grass. Look, it's getting long." Or, "We need to rake the leaves. Let's go." At first, I'd participate with him for five minutes, and then I was done. He would try his best to get me to do more and more. Kim would be at work, so just Ian and me would be at my old house. There used to be a waterbed in one of the rooms, and if I had my way, I'd lie on that bed snoozing all day. Of course, Ian would let me rest a little bit. We would have lunch, and I'd sleep—that was a routine. But he wanted me to be as active as I could be in the morning.

For months, Ian dragged me out there and I hated every minute of it. At last there was a turning point. Ian remembers that one day, Niko, Kim's dog, had dug some holes over by the farmhouse, and I said to Ian, right out of the blue, "Jeez, we gotta fill these holes in or someone's gonna break their ankle." And he thought, "This is fantastic!" First, that I was picking up on the problem, and second, that I was caring enough to do something about it. He stood back and watched in amazement as I went to the barn and got a shovel, got the wheelbarrow, went over to the garden, put three or four shovelfuls of dirt in the wheelbarrow, and went back to one of the holes that I'd found and filled it in. That was a huge breakthrough. It's funny, such a small thing. But Ian remembers it as the first time I really took an interest in anything. Without his encouragement and determination, I don't know if I ever would have gotten to that point.

It might have been another week before I was interested in doing something at the farm again, but being upset about those holes was an indication to Ian that there was something stirring around in me and changing for the better. Situations in which I successfully tackled minor but significant challenges became more frequent. I would rake the leaves for ten minutes instead of five, then fifteen and then twenty. We planted a garden in the first couple of years after my stroke, and Ian ended up doing 90 per cent of the work. But then I started to do more. He was always trying to steer me toward things I'd normally do, now that I was retired. He knew that if I hadn't had the stroke, I'd be spending time out there, so it made sense to get me to a point where I would want to do that again.

Socializing was another big challenge for me. I loved the guys I had worked with at Bell all those years. We'd had good times together at work, and playing hockey after hours in our younger years. Some of my friends were still working and some were retired. Ian used to take me over to Mister C's coffee shop on Thursday mornings, when the guys would get together for coffee. When I first started going, I was so uncomfortable that I didn't want to be there. Ian would buy me a coffee and donut, and we'd go over to sit with the guys. He wouldn't even have taken his seat when I'd be finished my coffee and donut and saying, "Okay, let's go." The guys would try to talk me into sticking around, but I'd say, "No, we've got to go." First couple of times he took me, we weren't there more than four minutes.

The thing was, I couldn't handle a social situation. Not even with old friends. I think it was because at those times, I was confronted with my deficits. I knew that I couldn't really contribute to the conversation, and I felt so lost. I had no way of relating to most of what they were saying to me. I was more comfortable staying in Ian's car, where I wouldn't have to confront that reality. The guys would say, "Hey Wally! Come on over," and want to joke and laugh and get me involved, but I just wasn't there yet.

For awhile, I hated Ian for doing this to me. "Why do you take me there all the time? What are we here for?" I'd say. I didn't understand that he wasn't trying to punish me, that he just wanted to gradually reintroduce me to these situations. I think it was Ian's persistence, and Phyllis's and Kim's—they simply didn't give up on me—that was important. They forced me to do things to the point where I was mad at them a lot, but it really worked out for the better. Eventually, I was not only happy to go out to meet my old friends for coffee, I couldn't get enough of it, or of any other social situation for that matter. But it took time for me to get to that stage, and everyone had to be patient with me while I struggled.

Ian viewed it as a sign of progress whenever he was able to fade out of the picture with me. Eventually, if we had a couple of things to pick up at Canadian Tire, he would give me a list, and I would go into the store by myself. Ian would wait in the car outside, right by the door, so he could see me coming out or run in if I got into trouble. Those were the little ways that I got my independence back. It was a big accomplishment for me to be able to go into a store by myself, buy items and come back out. Even I began to recognize that these were things I could and wanted to do for myself.

IAN: He's a survivor, a fighter. He has strong beliefs, and a lot
of this is ingrained in his own kids. That was something that
kept my hopes up. I knew that he was not going to give up.
Even those times when he wasn't all that motivated, he had
the grit and the drive to get better. That carried me through
his recovery, because I see a lot of people who just don't have
that. If you don't have it, it's easy to just lay down and die, to
give up. He never gave up on himself. He needed a lot of
encouragement at times. He was trying to make sense of his
own life. But he's always been the one saying that if you are
going to take something on, you should do it 110 per cent.
He's living proof—he took his own advice.

This whole experience was so difficult for Phyllis, it really was,
although she had terrific help. She and Kim are two peas in a pod,
and the relationship they have as mother and daughter is special.
They worked together as a team, Phyllis had never paid bills, and
she had to learn all of that. Kim helped her.

During my recovery, Phyllis was always interested in
doing the best for me. That was her main priority. But there
were times when she needed to get out of the house—she'd be
the first to tell you that. She had to deal with everything: the
kids, the grandkids, the whole world, her injured husband and
Ellen, too. I realize now that it was pretty emotionally tough
on her. There were days when Ian would pull in the driveway
and her car would already be running! She'd be gone, and I
don't blame her. But even so, she was always home to make
sure I had supper.

IAN: I think being Mr. and Mrs. Gretzky can be pretty challenging at the best of times. There were always a lot of pressures, and they didn't ease up after Wally's aneurysm—constant requests for autographs and appearances, people coming right to the door. All that was left to Phyllis. She had huge stress. But she always was there for Wally, always had great ideas for things to do with him. I might have been the guy who was showing up and being paid to work with her husband, but she made more suggestions than I did. She didn't just leave it up to me. She made sure Wally spent time with his friends, that the games were on, even if he wasn't all that interested, that Butch and Eddie were coming over to watch them with him. She had a sense this would help him in the long run, and she was right.

When I think about what Phyllis went through all those early years of my recovery, the thing I admire most is that she was never embarrassed to be with me, even when I was in very rough shape and didn't really know what was going on. This had to have been a challenge; she would have had to put herself in situations that were uncomfortable. Yet she would take me anywhere, any time. If we had to go to a wedding, we went. Or she'd take me up to Swiss Chalet for a meal. People would stare at us anyway, because of who we were. If I was looking a little bit sick, a little bit confused, you know, it might have been easier just to have stayed at home, but she never did. She would get me out of the house. She did that for me. She always made sure I had the opportunity to see my sons and their families, too. And I am sure that it was that strong attitude of hers that really helped me get back on my feet, as much as anything.

IAN: What was interesting about Wally was how well he did in public situations at that time. I mean, he was still quite disoriented, but he could do a television interview, as long as he was carefully prepared. One time, Glen arranged for Wally to be interviewed at Glen's apartment in Toronto. We said to the reporter, "Please do your best not to ask him questions about his current situation." His memory was that short. The reporter was great and asked things like, "How do you think Wayne is going to feel playing at the Gardens?" And I remember Wally's answer. This was a ten-minute interview. I swear to God, he turned it on! He was great. He talked about Maple Leaf Gardens, which he could, because that was knowledge that he still had. He knew Maple Leaf Gardens. He said, "As you know, Maple Leaf Gardens is a shrine. The history in that building . . . every time Wayne plays in that building, it really affects him emotionally. It's the first place he ever saw an NHL hockey game with his grandmother . . ." And I'm sitting back there in amazement, thinking, "Oh my God, this is wonderful." So he did a really good interview, his very first one. He was very brave. The reporter didn't put him on the spot. Because if you'd asked him two minutes later, "Who's playing?" he would not have been able to tell you.

Ian constantly drilled me with questions and memory exercises. Because I have always been a history buff, he got me quite interested in trivia, and I got into the habit of reading up on various historical facts and drilling other people. I guess I must have been a bit of a pain about it, but everyone was pretty tolerant of me grilling them! Our neighbour and friend Roly Bye still chuckles about it, because I'd walk into his house and just say, "I gotta ask you something." It would be a historical question or something to do with sports. "Do you know who scored three goals in twenty-one seconds?" He'd say, "Who?" I'd tell him it was the fastest three goals in NHL history: twenty-one seconds, Bill Mosienko, 1952, Chicago Blackhawks against New York. I met the guy who was Mosienko's winger. I played golf with him two years ago. The guy remembers the three goals. Do you know how they did it? They were all from faceoffs at centre ice. He'd be circling. The guy was a left-winger, and just as the puck was dropped, he'd be in full flight already. Today you can't do what he did then. Now you've gotta be stationary, you can't be skating around. That's how they did it, the guy told me.

After a few of these sessions, Roly's wife, Gloria, told him, "When Wally tells you something, you'd better mark it down, because he's going to come back again." Oh I did. I'd forget I'd already done the whole routine with them and come back the next day. The odd time, they'd remember the answer, and I'd say in amazement, "You knew that!"

I still love to quiz people, especially about history. But I can see that back then, this was just another way for me to build up some kind of organized memory and reach out to people in a way that I could control. I guess I knew I wouldn't get so confused or over-whelmed if I asked questions I knew the answers to.

When I started speaking in public, around 1995, I had made

a lot of gains, and my family felt confident of my ability to handle myself. But still, I needed a great deal of help. Ian remembers that after that interview about the Gardens, which had gone so well, I suddenly looked at him and asked, "Ian, where are we?" He told me we were in Glen's apartment in Toronto and explained why we were there. Then Phyllis came in, and immediately I wanted to know where Ellen was. Ian had to say, "Wally, you and I drove down here. We're going to see Wayne play a game tonight." He was still giving me reminders all the time.

It was tough. They'd take me to games at the Gardens, and unbeknownst to me, I'd be on *Hockey Night in Canada* all the time. The camera would pan around and find me, and Don Cherry would say, "Look, there's Walter Gretzky! Wally, it's great to have you back! Walter Gretzky is in the building!" And yet what no one knew was that throughout the games, as Ian sat with me, I would be whispering to him, "Where's Ellen? When's the game gonna be over?" And he would be whispering back, "Wally, just relax and watch the game." I still needed Ian as a mental walking stick at all times. He always wanted to help me look my best, but he was on pins and needles, never really knowing what might happen. He was always trying to keep two steps ahead of me, running interference if need be. People would approach me and say, "Hello Wally!" thinking that I was back 100 per cent, and Ian would have to redirect a lot of their questions or cue me, otherwise I wouldn't have a clue who they were or what they were talking about.

Over time, I learned how to cover my memory deficits in public situations, and now I can be comfortable most of the time. I'll always be polite to people when they approach me and tell me a story from the past, even if I don't remember it specifically. Of course, there were and are times when it can be frustrating, too. It's hard to hold up your end of the conversation when you haven't got the same reference points as the other person, and I would prefer to avoid those awkward moments. But I always try to say something anyway, because I know it means a lot to someone who has taken the trouble to come over and talk to me. I've been able to piece together the missing years from what others have told me and from looking at old photos that show me that particular things happened. It's the story of a part of my life that I can try to memorize and hold in my mind. If nothing else, I've learned to joke about my problems. I discovered that it is easier to be upfront about them than to try to hide them, and with that attitude, I can be comfortable dealing with most situations.

IAN: One thing that became a part of my job was travelling with Walter. Phyllis wanted him to go places, and she knew he needed an escort. So sometimes I'd arrive on a Monday morning and she'd say, "How would you like to go to L.A.?" Next thing you know, we'd be on a plane down there, and that evening, we'd be eating dinner with Wayne, Bruce McNall and John Candy! I must admit, I ended up in situations I never expected to encounter as a rehabilitation therapist! My friends got a great kick out of it. They'd say, "Hey, I saw you on Hockey Night in Canada last night!" Of course, it was all a lot of fun, quite amazing, really. Going to an L.A. Kings practice and meeting Wayne in the dressing room afterwards. Driving through Beverly Hills with Wally, Wayne and Janet—at times like that, I would often think, "What the heck am I doing here?" But it was good for Wally, and it gave Phyllis peace of mind to know that he could go places, and I was with him to make sure he didn't wander off or get into trouble. We went to Atlanta to see Brent play, and San Diego to see Keith. I got one of my first glimpses of how hard it was for Wayne while he was on the road. It was after a game at the Buffalo Auditorium, and the fans were just pushing up against the team bus, getting really frantic. Wayne was making a run for it, and I was behind him. Wally wasn't moving very fast in those days, so I was kind of dragging him along as fast as we could go. The security people were trying to push people back and Wayne was pleading with them, "I just want a couple of minutes alone with my dad. I just want to talk to my dad." They managed to have a bit of time together there, but then Wayne had to say, "Bye, Dad," and get on the bus. The fans were going insane.

There's no question I needed Ian to be with me most of the time, especially in public. But eventually, I became more confident when I was in a situation with strangers. I think my first public speech after the stroke was probably at Brent's wedding, when he married Nicole. Brent got married in June, 1995. I was pretty nervous, and my speech was very brief. But the more I spoke, the more I came to enjoy it. I had no idea back then that it would become something I'd be asked to do regularly, but it was the beginning of something that would grow to occupy a good deal of my life.

I would say that it was two and a half to three years after the aneurysm that I started to have some ability to be truly independent and to have enough short-term memory retention that I could start and complete a task. I cannot stress enough how important Ian's role was in getting me to this stage of healthy functioning. Even Dr. de Villiers, who, without a doubt, saved my life, has said that Ian's one-on-one therapy was the key to my recovery. And I should also point out that I realize how very lucky I was to receive it. We had the means to hire someone like Ian full-time; I'm fully aware that not everyone does, and that many people who could benefit from this kind of intensive long-term therapy do not receive it. But more and more, experts in the field of stroke and aneurysm are recognizing that the key to helping victims of these brain events to become thriving survivors is this level of attention.

By the time Ian was ready to wrap up his time with me, early in 1995, I finally understood that my mother had indeed passed away, that Brent was a grown-up and that I really was retired from my job at Bell. I was starting to piece together and accept what had happened to me, and was beginning to get the idea that with effort on my part, my life could move on. I had been taken off the medication they'd given me to help control my emotions, and suddenly, I had more energy, and more interest in being out and around people. I'd well and truly quit smoking; the original nicotine withdrawal had actually taken place, slowly and painfully, while I was in the hospital recovering from the surgery. Now I was nagging everyone else to give up the habit!

It was a step forward to be able to buy something at Canadian Tire on my own, do a few chores at the farm, attend a hockey game or talk to people at public functions, albeit under the watchful eye of Ian and members of my family. But now I had some drive of my own to get better—and some drive to, well, drive!

That was a big deal for me, getting my licence back. One of the first things that happens after a stroke like mine is that the authorities revoke your driving privileges, which is entirely justifiable. But I knew I'd feel far more genuinely independent if I could drive myself. We had to get the approval of the doctor before I could even have a driving test. The provincial testers had to be sure that I had the ability to pay attention, that I had good enough concentration and reaction time. They asked questions, and then they got me in the car and monitored every mistake. I missed a road sign, and they were concerned about that. They didn't give me my licence back right away. When I finally got it in February, 1995, I was proud of myself! If you get your licence back, it means you've made a pretty darned good recovery. The one lingering worry was that I drove too slowly and maybe couldn't handle driving at high rates of speed. Could I handle that much coming at me or would I try to slow it down too much? Driving is pretty much the most complex task that any of us do. Hundreds of decisions need to be made per second. I was driving way under the speed limit. But I told Ian, "I was trained. I drove the Bell trucks for thirty-five years and was told to drive five kilometres under the speed limit. Those people are wrong!"

Now I drive all over the place. Phyllis will say, "I need milk and bread. Can you drive to the grocery store and get it?" Sometimes I will still forget. I mean, we all do this. I'll leave and be gone for half an hour and come back with nothing and wonder, "What the hell was I supposed to get anyway?" I'll get to where I'm going, and somebody will start talking to me, and I will forget the items I was supposed to pick up. But I joke about it.

I was aware that I was getting more independent and needing Ian less. But other things were going on around me that I wasn't picking up on at the time, and it wasn't on account of my memory lapses. Life truly is full of surprises, and in this case, I'm delighted to say, it was a good one.

IAN: Kim and me. How did that happen? Well, I saw her so much when she came to see her dad. When Wally went home, and I was helping him, I saw her all the more. We formed a pretty close friendship. But we started to see each other as more than friends near the end of my working with Wally. Because of the close contact we had around him, I could see what a strong and caring person Kim was, and what a bond she had with her family. I think she saw that in me, too. I don't know, it really grew out of our close friendship. But neither of us wanted it to interfere in any way with Wally's recovery. When I left him to go back to work at the hospital, I guess I knew at that point I wasn't going to really be gone anyway! Phyllis already knew. I think I was so much a part of the family by then, nobody was surprised. I finished up full-time with Wally in February, 1995, and Kim and I got married in August.

But the biggest reason that we decided it was time was that we didn't want Wally to become too dependent on me. He sometimes had a tendency to let me do things that he really could do. When I wasn't around, he seemed able to do a lot more for himself. So I sat down with him and said, "You know, I think it's time for me to go." And he agreed to that.

I know Wally continues to deal with the memory deficits, but what's unique about him is that he's developed these coping tools, and he doesn't worry about it so much. He doesn't worry about small things any more, either. His focus is so much on other people anyway. He always had that compassion, but I think it's developed even more since the stroke. I think if I was meeting him for the first time today, I'd think, "What a great guy." I feel lucky to have spent the time I have with him. He is my role model. And my father-in-law!

They were married six months after Ian wrapped up his time as my official rehab therapist. Today, they live on the family farm, and have three young boys of their own. I have to say that I'm glad I didn't have two daughters, because I wouldn't have wanted to have two strokes in order to find them both husbands.

I can't say there was a particular day or moment when I realized I was truly getting better. It was literally years of hard work and gradual steps forward in my recovery before I was independent again. My friends and family say there were moments for them, too, when they realized, "Hey, Wally's getting better." For my buddy Bryan, it was the day he saw me driving in my own car up to his house. It shocked him, because he didn't even know I had my licence back! Now he says the only problem is that I forget to drive over and visit him often enough.

Keith and Wayne say they knew I was better when I started picking out my clothes again and got out of jeans and running shoes—items I'd never wear before!

BRENT: One of the big moments for me was when I was telling him about how I did in a game, and he said, "Well, did you get any goals?" And I said, "No, I got a couple of assists." For a long time, he just hadn't been interested. And then the next time he asked, I had gotten a goal and two assists, and we lost four-three, and he said, "Well, what happened to the second goal?" And I thought, "Oh, he's definitely getting better!" When he started talking about how 100 per cent of the shots won't go in, you know, and drilling me about it, we were all thinking, "He's getting better. He's getting back to himself." Yeah, when he started yelling back at us and giving us pointers on hockey, that was a good thing. I would call him on purpose and say I didn't do well during the games, just to hear his voice, just to hear him talk about hockey with me.

PHYLLIS: Oh, it seemed it went on forever, Wally's recovery. But when he went off all of his medication, we saw a big improvement. A lot of it he had to take, but as they gradually took him off it, he started to improve. It was a huge difference when the pills all stopped. But he is a totally different person.

KIM: Everyone will tell you, and it's true, that my dad's a different person now. Before the stroke, my dad did everything in the house. He paid the bills. He did all the man things! And my mum was—she was Mum. So for her, it was a time of adjustment. That was something that he always took care of. She was busy with the five kids at home. After the aneurysm she just had to deal with so much. She was wonderful to him.

His recovery was very gradual. As Ian says, you'd think you were making leaps, and all of a sudden, you'd be at a standstill. And then he'd progress again. Then he'd go backwards . . . but all these phases he had to go through. The stroke has changed him. In a lot of ways, good ways. He is so much less serious now. Sometimes we have to . . . well, my mum called one night and told Ian that she wanted a refund! I guess my dad had been carrying on, just being silly, which is nice to see, because for so many years, you never really saw that side of him. He's wonderful with little children. Absolutely wonderful with them. He'll pick my boys up at school and take them to McDonald's for lunch, which, my mum says, he never did with one of his own five children. The boys adore him.

GLEN: Really, he's two different guys. Before, he wouldn't miss a hockey game for anything. Now, he'll make sure he shovels four driveways before he watches TV. Before, not a chance. He's got way more energy now. I think it's just that whole "another chance to live" sort of thing. He has no sense of time. The best way to describe his behaviour is, you know, time doesn't exist. If he has to be somewhere at eight, but he's talking to someone, he won't leave until he's completely satisfied that he's talked to that person long enough. You have to understand that that's just the way he is. If you don't understand that, then it can be frustrating for you. He hasn't made a 100 per cent recovery, but he does incredibly well.

I think all of us have found our own ways of coping with Dad getting sick. I think about how it must affect Wayne, that Dad doesn't remember his records and Stanley Cups. And Keith, who was retiring from playing hockey and starting a new career in coaching without Dad's help. And Kim, who sacrificed three years of her life to look after not just my dad, but Mum and Ellen, too. And my dad not remembering that Brent was a teenager, and not being able to make it to Brent's NHL draft. And though we realize that Dad's not the same person now, we're all happy that he made it through and that we still have him as he is—which is wonderful.

Another twist along the road to recovery for me was finding out that I enjoyed playing golf. You have to know that this was quite a surprise to my family. Before my aneurysm, I had no time for the game. I thought it was stupid and said so. What could be more ridiculous than whacking a little round white ball around a big green lawn? Give me a wooden stick, a black rubber puck and some ice any day! I simply did not see the appeal. But once again, Ian was thinking about anything that I could possibly do with my time now that I was retired. Several of my friends golfed, so he arranged to have me go out with one of them. At first, I wasn't any more interested in participating in this than I was in anything else. But gradually I took to it. Now I can honestly say I love the game! When I'm home, I'm out three times a week with my friends Warren MacGregor, Bob Coyne and Burt Beney. Maybe it's because I'm moving around, and it helps me with my restlessness.

And maybe learning golf coincided with the time when I was becoming more social and outward-looking. Being out with my friends, sharing a laugh, walking around—really, it's perfect!

There are many things that I never imagined possible in my life, but one thing I genuinely never would have predicted was that I'd end up playing a game of golf with the man who saved my life. But several years ago, I found myself partnered at a tournament with Dr. de Villiers to raise money for a children's hospital. I was actually formally introduced to him, and I put my hand out and said, "Thank you ever so much, Doctor." It was the first time I really got to say that. I was in his office after the operation, but I have no memory of that.

All he said in reply was, "Don't thank me, it was your own will to live and everybody else who helped you." He's a very humble person.

When the golfing was over, there was a banquet at which I was supposed to speak, and we were seated together waiting for dinner. Dr. de Villiers leaned over and said in a soft voice, "By the way, Walter, there's an apology I want to make to you. I truly am sorry."

"What?"

"Well, when I operated on you I never expected it to happen, and I am sorry."

I jumped to the logical conclusion and said, "Don't worry, Doctor. Sure I don't have much of a memory, but no more headaches. I'm fine."

"Well, Walter," he said, "you might think you're fine, but I want you to know how sorry I am."

"What are you talking about?"

"Walter, when I opened you up, I never expected what happened."

By now, my heart was starting to pump, I could barely speak. I had to catch my breath. I said, "Please tell me what you're talking about."

"Well, Walter, when I opened you up, I wasn't truly prepared. I didn't realize there was so much intelligence in there, and it just poured out. I wasn't able to contain it all. You obviously understood what Einstein felt every day of his life."

"Doctor," I replied, hardly missing a beat, "I still can."

He's a great guy and one of the best surgeons around.

BOB COYNE: I remember when we had dinner with Dr. de Villiers at that golf tournament, and he leaned over the table to me and said, "You know, you cannot imagine how overwhelmed I am at this moment. Most of my successful patients are in wheelchairs in recovery homes somewhere, not speaking, just sitting. The unsuccessful ones, of course, don't make it at all. For me, walking in here tonight and witnessing this man speaking to a crowd the way I've just seen . . . I'm just not used to this."

It was very emotional for Dr. de Villiers to meet Wally. He was really moved and impressed.

Well, I am grateful for a lot of things, Dr. de Villiers's help among them. I truly knew I was recovering when I started to feel grateful. How could I not? So many people helped me out. I'm still in the process of trying to thank everyone.

For instance, I'll always remember the look on Laurie Ham's face about three years ago, when I showed up out of the blue at the Sheraton Hamilton Hotel, where she works as a corporate sales manager. I wanted to surprise her. She certainly wasn't expecting to see me, all those years later, standing in the lobby with open arms and a bouquet of flowers, but I did want her to know how much I appreciated what she had done for me, that day back in 1991. That was very important to me. And to show her, and maybe myself, too, just how far I'd come.

In many ways, these past few years have been the beginning of a whole new life for me, and I am as surprised and delighted as anyone else to have been given this kind of "second chance" gift. When people say there's no looking back, you can take it almost literally in my case. I'm not the man I was before 1991 and never will be. I accept that. But I'm not the man I was just after my aneurysm, either. I've moved on. Whatever my problems, something happened to me along the way to my recovery. Something good. Something that changed my attitude, my sense of myself, and turned my life into something once again worth living.

chapter six

BACK IN THE GAME

I really don't like to sit still for too long. I'm most comfortable when I'm active. I struggle day to day with long-term
memory loss and with short-term memory problems, but I've
developed techniques for remembering. I have to have ways to
cue my memory or I get into trouble. I went to the local Wal-Mart
in Brantford one day to get something for Phyllis. I parked the car
and then couldn't remember what I was supposed to bring
home. I went to the camera department and asked to use the
phone. I called Phyllis and said, "What was I supposed to get?"

It was embarrassing, even though the people who work in the camera department are friends of mine. When I came out, I was still so shaken up, I couldn't remember where I'd parked the blasted car. Wandered around, finally found it. Now if I go to the mall, I'll park in a certain spot, and count the lampposts from the car to the mall or look at where I am in relationship to the writing on the building. Am I under the letter "L" or the "T"? If I am going somewhere and doing more than one thing, I have a little notepad where I'll write it all down. That way, if I forget, I can always remind myself.

Of course, sometimes I forget to take my own advice. But people are always willing to help out if I can get over the embarrassment of asking for it. A couple of years ago I parked my car in downtown Brantford and neglected to write down some identifying landmarks. When I went to drive home, I couldn't find the car. I was standing there, scratching my head in frustration, when the mayor, Chris Friel, and a friend of his came walking along the street. I know and like Chris a lot, so I wasn't shy about telling him what my trouble was. He and his friend were concerned and kindly helped out, walking around the area with me until we finally found the car. Now these are young guys, in their early thirties, and I said, "Boys, don't ever have an aneurysm." That bit of fatherly advice cracked them up. Chris told me later that it has become something of a private joke between him and his friend. Whenever they can't find or remember something, they'll say to each other, "Boys, don't ever have an aneurysm." I don't mind them having a laugh about it—but I would seriously advise anyone not to have an aneurysm!

To this day, although I have enough memory to allow me to be independent, if you ask me for specific information about something that happened last week, I may not be able to tell you very accurately. What's common for all of us is that we remember significant events, but not so much the everyday things, which we don't consciously commit to memory. If somebody asked you what you had for dinner three nights ago, you probably couldn't remember right away. But if you thought about it, you could maybe make some associations. You'd say to yourself, "Okay, where was I?" And you'd start to build a picture, and eventually you'd come up with the answer. In my case, I'm not able to do that as well. But if a meteor was to fall out of the sky, I'd remember every detail of it, because like everyone, I remember more dramatic, out of the ordinary things. I'm pretty good that way.

It's a strange feeling, not being able to remember large parts of my life, but I've learned to live with that. I accept that sometimes strangers will come up to me and tell me that we met, and I just have to take their word for it. My family and friends are tireless in orienting me if a situation arises where that's necessary. I just listen to what people tell me, and try my best to place it in my memory, hoping that people will make allowances when they meet me.

I sleep fine now, but I still don't go to bed until the wee hours. I have always been a night owl. When there's no one else to phone or visit, I'll finally sit down on the couch and watch something on TV. I'm a real history buff, so I love to watch the History Channel. If something interesting is on, I'll watch TV till two in the morning. Half the time, I'll fall asleep on the couch, then wake up and go to bed. That's what I used to be like. Because of the time difference between here and L.A. or Edmonton, I would usually call Wayne in the middle of the night. Or I'd be in my office, looking through the fan mail at three in the morning. I'd go to sleep for a few hours, and then I'd have to get up and go to work. That just became a way of life, and not the healthiest one, I now realize.

I find it hard to believe some of the things people tell me about the early days after my stroke. Those were dark times, and I wouldn't want to go back there for anything in the world. It's an awful thing not to know who or where you are, to feel confused and hopeless and not know whether you are ever going to be able to do all the things you used to do. Everybody wants to be independent. Something simple that I would have taken for granted before, like driving, I had to accept that I would have to learn how to do all over again, along with all those daily routines and tasks that make you feel in control of your own life. It was independence and a sense of self-worth and purpose that I fought so hard to get back, even when I wasn't conscious of it.

I know now how much my loved ones wanted me to have my independence and sense of self-worth back, too, and how hard they all tried to help me. It wasn't easy for them, because, as you have read, I was in a pretty sorry state. But my family, with Ian's help, was determined to get me actively involved in the world again and really put a lot of effort into thinking of things for me to do. With their help and encouragement, I've come a long, long way.

Along with all the other things that helped me, I suppose it shouldn't come as too much of a surprise that hockey would finally play a significant role in my recovery.

Two years after the stroke—I remember that Ian was still with me—Phyllis got in touch with Peter Jones, who was president of the Brantford Minor Hockey Association at the time, and asked if there was a program they could get me into. She wanted me integrated back into the community, doing something I once loved, with kids. Peter called Bob Coyne, who said, "Well, I've got this little tyke program, four- and five-year-olds, and we're simply teaching them to hockey skate. I'll bet he'd have a great time with that. Let's do it."

So we did. But as Ian and Bob will tell you, when I first arrived at the rink, I didn't want to go on the ice. I didn't even want skates on. Ian and Bob had to put them on me. I said, "No, you guys go ahead. I'll just sit here and watch." I wanted to hide from the world, and I was miserable. Whatever love of hockey I once had, it was pretty much dead, or at least buried a long way down inside, and I had no desire to try to get it back. They'd insist: "No, Wally, you gotta go on the ice, let's go." They encouraged me, and eventually they got me on the ice.

I must admit, I enjoyed it just a little bit, even if I did have to be pushed. But I noticed right away that times had changed. It made me laugh to hear those little guys calling me Wally. I got such a kick out of that. In my day, an adult was always addressed as Mister or Sir or Coach. We would never have used his first name! I could not believe that, and it hit my funny bone. The kids would just pipe up, "Hey Wally, what are we doing next?" And that would make me laugh every time. At first, I think Bob and Ian were puzzled as to what exactly was amusing me so much, but they finally figured it out.

Eventually I started having lots of fun with the kids, but I'll tell you something I didn't like, and don't like to this day, and that's the behaviour of some of the hockey parents. Times have changed there, too. Sometimes it seems that minor hockey is no longer about the kids but about the parents, and that's wrong. I don't think you can teach a kid good hockey skills when the parents are interfering or skating around the ice themselves. Sometimes there were so many parents out on the ice during those Timbits practices, it was totally chaotic. I thought it was awful. It really upset me. I didn't like the parents telling the kids things that were absolutely against developing good skating skills, or pushing them to be the next Wayne when at that stage, especially, they should be on the ice having fun. It bothered me so much to see the kids not being taught the correct way to do things, that I wanted to back out of my commitment. Whatever else I'd lost with the stroke, one thing that seemed to remain intact was my sense of what's good for kids when they're learning how to play hockey. If we were going to be interfered with at every turn, I couldn't see the point.

But I didn't want to disappoint Bob. I said to Ian, "You tell Bob, I'm not coming tomorrow. I hate it. I'm not going out there." And Ian, of course, told Bob, and I guess they chuckled, but they thought, "We've got to keep him going. He can't stop." So finally, Bob asked Ian what it was that I really didn't like. And Ian told him, "It's the parents." You know, teaching their kids to step over sticks, when they can't even hold their balance on skates.

Stepping over the sticks forces their heads down, which is counterproductive. The other thing that really bothered me was the mess! I like to see a dressing room clean before I leave. All I have to do is walk into a room after a team has been there, and if it's a mess, I know the kids don't listen. I know the coaches aren't giving them discipline. So I like to stay right to the end. As much as you tell kids to clean up after themselves, they're going to leave things around—they're kids, for heaven's sake. But I like to tidy things up so that the next coach who comes in has a nice clean room. I really believe strongly in that. It's part of good sportsmanship to be as disciplined off the ice as you are on it.

BOB COYNE. I really wanted Walter to remain involved, and not just as team janitor—he is quite obsessed about picking up every last bit of tape in a dressing room and leaving the place spotless for the next team. Phyllis and Ian wanted him to keep going, for his sake and for the kids. We could see the potential for good there. So I said, "Okay, I'll go to my hockey group and say, 'No more parents on the ice.'" And you know what? It was the best thing we ever did. We got the parents off the ice, and Wally came out of himself incredibly. Then, he had a few things to say! It took off like wildfire. And that was the last of him wanting to quit. Five or six weeks after we banned the parents, you could see that he belonged to hockey again.

Just to reinforce the point with parents, I often read this poem when I speak to groups involved with minor hockey:

Please don't scream, curse or yell
Remember, I'm not in the NHL
I'm only nine years old
And can't be traded, bought or sold.
I just want to play the game
I'm not looking for hockey fame
Don't make me feel I'm made of sin
Just because my team didn't win.
I don't want to be so great, you see
I'd rather play and just be me
So always remember this little quip
The name of the game is sportsmanship.

(author unknown)

I like to remind parents, when they go to the rink or ballpark, and find themselves hollering at their son or daughter because they're not playing very well and the team is losing, to stop and think how lucky they are. Their child has got two eyes, two arms and two legs. Then I say, "Come with me at Christmastime and see the kids I visit in the hospital." We so often take for granted what a blessing it is to have healthy children, period, capable of playing a sport at all and benefiting from what there is to learn and enjoy when they do that. Many kids are not so lucky, and I have met enough of them to know.

Once Bob got the parents off the ice and me really involved, he decided that I needed to coach older kids, too. So he applied to the Brantford Minor Hockey Association and said he'd like to take the Triple A novice team the next year, and that he wanted me to help him. They said "By all means, it's all yours." I really did think of myself as Bob's helper and was quite willing to stay in the background. But then Bob strategically failed to show up for one of the tournament games, and there I was by myself, surrounded by a bunch of nine-year-old kids, all wondering what they were supposed to be doing. The littlest guy, the goalie, finally piped up: "So Wally, what's our starting lineup?" I looked around at those keen, questioning young faces and had to say something. I guess it was a bit like turning on a light bulb, because from then on, I didn't need any prodding from Bob, Ian or anyone else.

The following September, we coached the Triple A novice team again, and we had just a great time. I loved telling stories to those little guys, and of course they'd be there with big eyes, staring at me from the bench, figuring they'd better listen, because this is Wayne Gretzky's dad! Their enthusiasm reconnected me to the sport I love.

That year, we were in the first round of playoffs against Niagara Falls. That team had only just made the playoffs, and Bob and I had *the* team to beat. We were favoured to win the whole works. So the first round is the best of three, and we beat Niagara Falls in two. They're little kids, and they don't all handle defeat very well. On the night we eliminated them, the scene was cheerful in our dressing room. But as Bob and I were leaving, we encountered a few of the Niagara Falls kids. One little guy was standing beside his dad's car just crying his heart out. I stopped. Bob wanted to keep on walking. He's seen a lot of kids having a hard time. You understand in the hockey world that that's part of growing up, and this kid wasn't even on our team. But I said, "Bob! Bob, look at that little guy." And he said, "Wally, you don't have to deal with it." And I said, "Deal with it! He's a baby, for heaven's sake!"

I went up to the boy and said, "What's your problem?" knowing full well what his problem was.

He wailed, "Well, we lost!"

And I said, "But there's more to hockey than winning and losing. Did you have a good time?"

"Um, well, yeah."

"Well, that's all there is to it. Now, little guys like you oughta have a reward for working hard. Did you work hard?"

"Oh, I worked really hard."

"Well, see, that's all that matters. Now, where's the rest of your team?"

"They're still in the dressing room, but they're coming out."

I said, "Bob, go tell the rest of those kids in the dressing room, they're coming to my house, right now, to see Wayne's sweaters and the trophies."

Bob was a little taken aback by this, but he went in there. Of course they were not expecting him. He said, "Hi, I'm the coach from the other team. Walter Gretzky would like all of you, mums, dads, everybody, right now, to come to his house on Varadi Avenue, to see the trophy room." They all looked at him like, is this guy serious? They said, "Really?" He said, "Yes! Absolutely, right now. We're gonna convoy you out of here so we don't have to give you directions. Everybody follow everybody else, and we'll just meander right over there."

Bob says he never saw a dressing room clear so quick in all his life. Everybody was out in the parking lot, throwing gear into their cars, still thinking this wasn't really happening. I said, "Okay, follow us. Let's go, it's not very far from here." And we went. The head count going in the door at home was sixty-one. Poor Phyllis. She'd been expecting only Bob and me, and we arrived with sixty-one people! Not that that hadn't happened before . . .

> BOB COYNE: We took those little guys down into the basement, and that's really the essence of Wally, beaming at those kids putting on Wayne's sweaters and trying on Wayne's hockey medals, all sorts of things. I can remember one father standing there in awe, and he reached out to shake Wally's hand, and he said, "You know what? This is better than winning the all-Ontario championships. I can't think of a more fitting thing for these little kids." Wally just smiled at the guy, as though to say, "Well, this is what hockey ought to be all about, isn't it?" Very unassuming, that's his nature. Like, this has been no big deal. But those people from Niagara Falls, they had just died and gone to hockey heaven.

I love to see people's faces when they come down the basement stairs and look at some of this stuff. But, eventually, we had to curtail the number of people coming into the house. We had so much stuff in the basement, we figured it really deserved to be shown more formally. In 1999, the year Wayne retired, we shipped a lot of it to the Hockey Hall of Fame in Toronto, where they put together a fabulous display in honour of his induction there. They tell me it is a real hit. When I hear that, I am so glad I took the time to save all that stuff. I know Wayne is thrilled with it, too. As a kid, he certainly spent his share of time down at the old Hall of Fame, staring at the display cases of memorabilia from all the hockey greats. I'm sure there's a future NHL star or two doing the same thing there today. In fact, one of the nicest things about the induction ceremony was that Michael, the grandson of our long-time neighbours Mary and Sil, got to represent Wayne as a kid, wearing his original Nadrosky Steelers sweater. It's great when life sort of comes full circle like that. I treasure that memory.

Another memory I treasure is of a time I acted in a way that was maybe not too wise. One evening a few years ago, before all the trophies and mementoes went to the Hockey Hall of Fame, I came back from the arena and pulled into the driveway. It was around seven or so and not dark yet. There was a van parked on the street in front of our house, but I didn't pay much attention to it. When I got out of my truck, the driver came up to me and said, "Mr. Gretzky, is it okay if the guys get out and have a picture taken with you on your front lawn?" As usual, I said yes. Then I looked at the van and saw "Ministry of Correctional Services" on its side.

I forget how many young men there were, maybe eight or so. They got out of the van and had their pictures taken with me, individually and as a group. They were teenagers, basically, from about sixteen to twenty-one years old. I said, "You wanna come in and see the trophies?" Of course they said yes. So I took them all in and trooped them down to the basement.

Phyllis was upstairs. She wasn't having a bird—she was having about a dozen of them.

Anyway, when it was all over with, I stood in the driveway and they all lined up in order to shake my hand. I noticed one guy, who was first or second in line, drop out and go to the very back of the line. I wondered what he was doing. One thing I've learned from Wayne is to always be aware of your surroundings. So I noticed that. This guy was the tallest in the group, which is one of the reasons I noticed him. Anyway, as each young man went by, he shook my hand, said thank you and then headed for the van, which the guard had gone ahead to unlock. Finally, the tall young guy came through. He was the very last one. I took his hand to shake it, and he said thank you, but then, all of a sudden, he just started to cry. I mean, he was sobbing, and I realized why he'd gone to the back of the line. He didn't want the rest of them to see him in tears. He squeezed my hand and said, "Thank you, Mr. Gretzky. You would take us into your house, knowing who we are, where we are from? You would do that?" I said, "Well, you're no different than anyone else, for heaven's sake." And he said, "I'll remember this for the rest of my life. Nobody has ever done anything like this for me." And he just kept squeezing my hand. I'll always remember that.

Whenever I speak, I tell that story. People always clap. That's the part that surprises me, that people should think this was somehow out of the ordinary, rather than just the kindness we owe to each other, especially the troubled kids among us. I often wonder where that kid is, how he's doing. I wish him well.

Back to hockey. That first year when Bob and I went with our team to the all-Ontario finals, I went to the games all through the next series, bringing special pucks that Wayne had scored significant goals with and I visited the opposition's dressing room prior to each game. I usually didn't have to introduce myself. Each of the kids would get to touch Wayne's medal before a game, or see a puck that he scored a famous goal with. We were eventually knocked out, but that was okay. It was a wonderful, wonderful year.

BOB COYNE: Wally forced all of us to grow, because he's always thinking of other people. A typical scene when you go with Wally to the rink: If the game starts at seven and it's a little kids' game, it's over at eight, and you're leaving the arena at 8:30. With Wally, forget that. When he leaves the dressing room, he goes to the lobby. If somebody needs a picture for their grandfather, it's "here, give me your address and I'll get this to you." If someone needs an autograph on the spot, he's there for that. We don't leave that arena until he's satisfied that all the needs are met.

When I first got involved with Wally, I had a time frame. Like most people, I think I've gotta be home by a certain time, you know? But you come to realize very quickly, if you're going to continue your friendship with Wally, there are no time frames. If that's a problem, well, you just couldn't hang around him any more.

I don't lose track of time deliberately, you know, but it is true that since my stroke, my sense of time has altered. I don't like to keep people waiting, and I try not to, but I also can't stand the thought of someone coming to an event and wanting an autograph and having to leave without one. I think it's more a question of priorities for me. I like to make time for people. If someone wants to chat for a minute or two, get a photo and something signed, well, I don't have a problem with that. These people are the reason I'm in the fortunate position I'm in, and I never forget that.

In 1995, Bob and I were asked to coach the all-star game at the Cambridge minor hockey tournament in January. This is one of the biggest hockey tournaments in this part of Ontario for little guys, novices and atoms. In the middle of the tournament, they have an all-star game. They pick the best kids from the tournament, put them into two teams and they play each other. Now it's a highlight of the Cambridge tournament. They advertise it: "Walter Gretzky coaches the all-star team." You get kids there from all over Ontario, Michigan, New York State, Illinois. That all-star game is maybe more important to those kids than the tournament itself. You get some talented players, and we work to get them playing as a team. They're all motivated to do well for themselves, but we emphasize the need to work with their fellow players—it's not about being a star or hogging the limelight. When we go into the dressing room, I always make sure I've got a really good Wayne story to tell them. I'll explain to them what it took for Wayne to get where he is, all the practicing he did, the focus he had, and how if they work like him, they too can find that kind of success. That just seems to pump up the game.

WARREN MacGREGOR: I really believe that a lot of Wally's coaching theories are instinctive. He doesn't know why he wants you do something, but he knows it works. And that comes from his own hockey abilities. When Wally was young, he was a pretty slippery centre himself. His timing is just what he has taught Wayne. His idea of anticipating plays, it was the same thing. So a lot of what Wally does, he does from instinct. He knows it works. He's been there, he's done it.

More than anything, I want the kids to know that if you really believe in yourself, you can do anything you want. This is not just a nice sentiment. I try to give them reasons to believe in themselves. If a kid comes off the ice and has done well, it's important to go over and acknowledge it, in the right way for that moment. You don't want to be overenthusiastic or not enthusiastic enough. I know what a kid is looking for in terms of feedback about his playing, and when he (or she—I've coached girls, too) comes off the ice, I try to provide it. I also try to give a kid a sense of direction. For example, I'll tell him the goal was great, but next time, add this to it. Let the kid know that his way was the right way, but he could do more. Rather than saying, "Oh well, that was nice, but next time do it my way," I say, "Next time, do it your way again, but add more to your own way." You have to coach a kid to be himself. As a coach, you can't make clones of yourself. This kind of coaching was the secret of success for Wayne. Because of his body size, because of his weight and so many things, he could only pattern his game on himself. You had to recognize that and develop him to his best potential. I do that same thing with kids now.

Bob and I have also become very involved in the Challenge Cup in Burnaby, British Columbia. It's run by Billy Doherty, who also runs the Banff Hockey Academy in Alberta. This is one of the larger hockey tournaments in British Columbia, and it's held over a five-day period at a place called Burnaby 8-Rinks. There are literally eight rinks under one roof, and they boast on the sign in front of the arena that it's the largest hockey facility in the world. We always have a wonderful time there. I end up signing autographs from sun up to sun down.

As the tournament comes to a close each year, the organizers scurry me from one rink to another as championship games are played so that I can present the gold, silver and bronze medals. Sometimes games are actually held up because I'm doing a presentation on the rink. They really seem to want it to be me who places those medals around the players' necks. It's quite a panicky kind of affair on the last day. But we all enjoy ourselves, and I look forward to seeing the people involved each year.

Participating in these hockey tournaments and other events has become a huge part of my life over the past several years. My family and friends think maybe I've gotten too busy for my own good, but it doesn't feel like that to me. I'm happy to be busy, and grateful that I can be of service to others. Phyllis is great at monitoring everything, and she makes sure I don't overdo it too much, though I don't know how to relax and never have. I'll go out to the farm, where Kim and Ian now live with their three little boys, and start fixing things, and they'll say, "Take a couple of days off! Go to bed!" But I like to keep going.

The big change since the stroke is that though I'm still on the run all the time, I'm more happy-go-lucky about it. Not worrying about Wayne's hockey career certainly makes me a less nervous person all around! In some ways, the stroke helped me re-examine my priorities. I guess it has been a process of letting go, not just for me but for my loved ones, too.

KIM: Dad did then, and does now, instill respect into all of us. We were taught to show respect for ourselves and others. One of his big lines was always, "Never burn a bridge, in case you have to cross it one day." That kind of influence hasn't changed. But he doesn't have the same routines. Before his aneurysm, he spent a lot of time at the farm, while my grand-mother was alive and then after her death. I think he used to come out here just to get away, and he loved to be outside. He grew up here, and this is his home. He doesn't really come out the way he used to. He loved to fish before, and now he rarely goes fishing. He would come here and fish for hours. He still likes to do it, but he doesn't so much any more.

BRYAN WILSON: He was always telling me he was a better fisherman than me, or that I shouldn't do this or that, you know, in a nice, jokey way. I miss that. I miss Walter phoning me up and saying, "Where are you? The game's started!" And if I'd say, "Oh I don't feel like going out tonight," he'd say, "You get your ass over here." It's just all those old times you miss when you're close friends with someone. Now he's so busy, he forgets he's supposed to come and visit me! What he does with kids is just great. I'm happy he's alive, and happy to see him do all this stuff. But I'll admit I sometimes wish I could talk to him or go fishing like we used to.

WAYNE: Within my family, we know the differences in Dad. We've encouraged him to pick up his camera, but he's just not interested. This is the guy who watched me play hockey for thirty-six years, never missed a game or practice if he could help it from the time I was little. That's gone, but I think he's got more peace of mind now. He's still got his passion for life. I'd say he's a happier person today. Not that he was unhappy before—it's just . . . a different kind of happy.

I understand that sometimes they all miss the guy I was. Maybe they can't talk to me in quite the same way as they used to. On the other hand, I know everyone is grateful I survived and pleased that I can enjoy life now in a way I seemed less able to before. I never really gave myself the chance. But now that I'm retired and recovered, and have so few worries in the world, everything I do seems optional and a lot of fun, not a burden or responsibility.

BOB COYNE: Every year in Burnaby, he's pounding on my door at the crack of dawn, "Bob, Bob, let's go, gotta get down to the rink!" And I'm like, "Wally, it's 6:30, nobody's there yet!" And he's "No, no, gotta get some breakfast, we gotta be there." We'll get into the car and down we'll go to the rink, and there'll be a few early birds. And as soon as they see him, wow, there's a mob around him. I don't know where they come from. That's early, early in the morning. And that mob will still be there late at night. I'll almost have to get mad at them to get rid of them. Sometimes he'll give me a look like, that's nasty. Sometimes you have to play the role of the bad guy, just to protect Wally, just to let him get some lunch. If I didn't break it up, he'd stand there all day, and just sign and tell stories and have a good time with people until he collapsed. And they love him. They just love him to death.

Some amazing and wonderful things happen when I'm out meeting people. I recall a time two or three years ago in British Columbia when I was signing autographs and the line was really long. Bob became aware of a man standing off to my right with tears coming down his face. The man noticed that Bob was looking at him, and he came over and asked Bob whether he was with me. Bob said he was, and the man asked, "Are you the guy who worked at the school for the blind in Brantford?" And Bob said that yes he was.

"Well, my grandson has just had an operation. They've removed his eye," the man said. "He lost his other one a year ago. Now he's totally blind. And I heard about Walter Gretzky working with blind kids." He was crying again. "What am I going to do with my grandson? He's got no eyes."

I finished up with autographing, and Bob introduced me to this gentleman. He told me the situation, and I got all choked up. He wanted an autograph for his grandson, so we got out an eight-by-ten of Wayne and I signed it. When I got home, I sent some more stuff out for this little boy.

The next year, I had to go out to Prince George for a speaking engagement. As coincidence would have it, the boy was from Prince George, and I went to see him. He was just so thrilled. I've kept in contact, and every once in a while, I get to say hi to him in person. Those are the kinds of great things that happen to me all the time.

Once I got my interest in hockey back, there was no stopping me. In 1996, Bob and I were looking for something to do in the summer, and we got involved with in-line hockey. That was quite a change. An opportunity had come up for us in Brantford to coach a bunch of little house-league kids called Rolling Thunder. We thought, "Why not? We don't know a thing about the sport, but we'll have fun." And we had a great time. We kind of guessed our way through the whole thing, and since the kids were little, it wasn't too hard to fool them!

These kids really didn't have a whole lot, and they were not really athletes, but they were very receptive to coaching. When we first took the team over, roller hockey was something they did if they weren't doing anything else on Saturday morning. As we went on, it got to be a big deal if they had to miss a practice. The fun to be had was worth coming for. Here Bob and I were, not knowing anything about this game, and our team got right down to the championships, simply because we tried to make each of those kids feel that the team needed them, they had to be there and it didn't matter how good they were. Once they had tried their best, it was okay with me. I accepted them, and that was a great lesson for them. You don't have to be the best to be accepted by me. But I will know if you haven't tried your best, and you will know I know—just ask any of my kids! It doesn't matter what the sport is or the level of play, the same principles for success apply.

The next year we went from the sublime to the ridiculous. Here we were, the first time we'd ever coached the sport with a bunch of little kids playing house-league roller hockey, and the next season we went right to Major Junior A. That was quite a step up, from little seven- and eight-year-olds to kids between seventeen and twenty-one playing at the elite level. It was the league's first year of operation, and there were teams from all over southwestern Ontario involved: all the kids who had been playing casually, or had played hockey in the winter and wanted a fun but challenging summer sport. Bob was asked to be on the organizing committee. They had to decide how they would determine the championship, who the cup would be named after, all of that. Bob put my name forward for the championship trophy. So the cup we played for that year was the Walter Gretzky Cup.

Our team was the underdog all season, simply because neither Bob nor I knew much about the game. But it seemed to me that Wayne's style of hockey lent itself perfectly to roller hockey. Deviation as opposed to domination. Anticipating where you should be and being there before your opponent knows what's going on—not fighting your way to the goal. That's my whole philosophy now on roller hockey. My aim is to teach the kids how to be other than what they are opposing. If you can't be the biggest and the strongest and the toughest, you can simply be the smartest. It worked for Wayne. Understand where the play's going, and be there. We didn't worry about whether we had the six-foot-two guys, as long as we had a five-foot-seven guy with a lot of heart, great speed and a good brain.

And you know what? It worked. We went into the championship game against Mississauga, and into the last minute we were trailing by a goal. Then one of their players was knocked unconscious, and the game was delayed for half an hour while the ambulance came to take him to hospital. As a result, we had a man advantage, and we scored, tying the game with something like twenty-two seconds left. At 8:02 of sudden death overtime, we won the Walter Gretzky Cup. Those who are into hockey know that 802 is very special to Wayne. That was the goal that broke Gordie Howe's record of 801. When the boys scored the winning goal, I was sure the gods were on our side. It was a wonderful day.

There's a kids' ice hockey tournament named after another Gretzky: the Wayne Gretzky International, which happens every year at the end of December. I'm what you might call a fixture there, and over the years, I've done a whole lot of presenting to the kids and the coaches. Well, last December, I got to be on the other side of the medal ceremonies with the hockey team I coached with Bob. It was a storybook thing, because we were not even considered contenders going into that tournament. But we won our first game, and Bob said, "Wow." Then we won our second game, and he said, "I don't think I believe this." And then we won our third game and he said, "No, I'm in a dream. This can't be happening." The kids just jelled and they played their hearts out. As little as they were.

BOB COYNE: Going into that game, I made sure the boys knew that Wally had never won a Wayne Gretzky medal, and that became our obsession. I'd say, "Kids, we gotta do this. We can't go in the penalty box. We gotta play for each other. No hot dogs in this game, we've got to play like we're a team. If ever we've been a team, today we are going to be a team." And we won the championship in our division. You should have seen Wally, it was unbelievable. He was so happy. Then the big joke came at medal time: who presents the medal to Wally, since Wally presents the medals?

Moments like that one are precious to me, and there were many of them while I was coaching those kids. But at the end of the season last year, I retired from coaching. With so many other involvements, it was starting to be something I couldn't put all my energy into, and that's not fair to the kids. Coaching is a big responsibility, in my opinion, and you have to be fully committed to it if you are going to do it at all. And to be honest with you, I'm still not impressed with the way many of the parents conduct themselves, and that really takes away from the fun of the game. Now I'll have more time to go to the rinks whenever I want and keep doing all the other things I enjoy, as well. I'll still be on hand to give out medals, sign autographs at tournaments, drop the odd puck and offer bits of advice here and there when I'm asked. Without doubt, being with the kids and watching them do well, maybe better than they or anybody else thought they could, are among my happiest memories from my recovery.

BOB COYNE: In the very beginning, it was an honour to be asked to work with Walter Gretzky. I'm not much different than other people—I was thrilled! Wow. But along the way, he's become a good friend. I'd die for the guy. His ability to recover, to surge forward and be something is very special. We, as Canadians, have a little bit going for us in the world: no one else has Walter Gretzky. Do you know Babe Ruth's dad's name? Gordie Howe's dad's name? I mean there is a unique quality to Walter.

IAN: It's amazing to consider how unmotivated and withdrawn Wally was in the beginning of his recovery, when it came to getting out and being with people. Now, you can't get him out of the rink or the coffee shop. He's gone to the other extreme. Whenever you go to a function with him, people have to kick him out at the end of the night. He just loves to be around people, to entertain, to tell stories. He loves to go to the rink just to hang around. He goes into the dressing rooms of out-of-town teams, and he's "Mr. Gretzky." He'll go from dressing room to dressing room, and the coaches are as much in awe as the kids are. He'll go in there and tell them a couple of stories about Wayne, or he'll say how important it is to listen to your coach. This is only part of what he does. His contribution to the community now is unbelievable.

chapter seven

REACHING OUT TO OTHERS

I guess I've always been oriented toward helping people wherever I can, looking out for those who are less fortunate. Maybe having a little sister with Down's syndrome gave me my awareness of the need for this, I don't know. All I know is that now that I've been given another chance at life, I feel even more motivated to give where I can.

For a long time before my stroke, my whole family was involved with the Canadian National Institute for the Blind, fundraising through the tournaments. I am particularly proud of two successful initiatives I am involved with in association with the CNIB. The first is the SCORE program (Summer Computer Orientation Recreational Education), which Wayne and I started in 1985. The camp was designed to assist and train exceptional blind and deafblind students in computer skills necessary for future careers and education, and to increase the students' access to the Internet and computer programs. So far SCORE has helped provide over five hundred career positions for past students.

As well, in 1995 I founded the Wayne and Walter Gretzky CNIB Scholarship for Blind and Deafblind Canadian students. I had never realized that the majority of blind students were unable to pursue post-secondary education due to a lack of finances—and that scholarships for blind students did not exist. So I decided to do something to help. The CNIB handed out the first scholarships in 1996, when three students received $5,000 each. In 2001 we gave out fifteen $5,000 scholarships. For both SCORE and the scholarship program I remain involved by helping with fundraising, as well as personally presenting awards and speaking with students who receive them.

We have a school here in Brantford called the W. Ross Macdonald School, for visually impaired kids, and they ask me to come and speak at their graduation ceremonies and hand out awards to their outstanding student athletes, and I am honoured to do it. And wouldn't you know, it was through hockey once again that I got involved in another very special project to benefit the school and other charities.

A couple of years ago, I was going through the school's shop department on a tour, when I saw a bench the students had made entirely from hockey sticks. I thought, "What a great idea." There's so much waste in North America, and it seems a shame to throw out good pieces of wood whenever a hockey stick breaks, which happens a lot over the course of a season. The bench was a sturdy piece of furniture. You could stand and jump on it, and it was even comfortable to sit on. I asked the instructor, Mel Andre, how they came to make it. He said the original idea came from a staff member who had seen a picture in a magazine. Her son was really into hockey, so she asked Mel if they could make a bench like the one in the picture. It took a few tries, but they finally came up with a design that worked. Mel and his students wanted to make more, but they couldn't get enough sticks. If people wanted a bench, Mel asked them to bring in forty-eight broken sticks. It takes twenty-four to make a bench, so with forty-eight they could make two; one for the person who had commissioned it, and one to give away as a fundraiser.

That got me thinking. I went around to some rinks, and everyone I talked to was happy to supply me with my first donation. Within a week, I had a carload of broken sticks. I mean, the back seat of the convertible was crammed full in every direction. I'm surprised I didn't puncture the roof—there would have been hell to pay with Phyllis if I had. But after I made my delivery, the school had enough sticks to make me a bench and a few more besides.

Now, collecting broken sticks is a part of my regular routine. Once a week or every two weeks, I go to the school's shop with a delivery. I visit the different rinks around the Brantford and Cambridge area, and they save all their broken sticks for me. You'd be amazed at what the students make from these hockey sticks that used to get thrown in the garbage. So far, they've made

105 benches. And they've expanded to other pieces of furniture as well: footstools, coffee tables, end tables, coat racks. They ask me to sign the top stick of each piece and they're used to fundraise all across the country. For instance, a little Manitoba town of about one hundred, including cats and dogs, with a gas station, general store and skating rink, was having trouble keeping the rink open and was looking for a way to fundraise. The school shipped a bench out there.

Mel says they can't keep up with the demand for the benches now. People auction them off. Big Brothers in Kitchener sold one in a charity auction for $2,550. So far, that's the record. The average winning bid is about $500. The school has donated about sixty of the one hundred they've made, and raised about $30,000 for other charities. The benches have sold all over Ontario, from Windsor to Ottawa, and west to Manitoba and Saskatchewan.

They'll keep making furniture as long as I bring in the sticks. They've got a set numbered ninety-nine that includes a table and bench, and one day, Wayne is going to sign that. Fifty to sixty students in grades seven to twelve are involved in building these benches.

DON NEALE, PRINCIPAL, W. ROSS MACDONALD SCHOOL: The very last day of school two years ago, at four o'clock, the students and staff had all gone home and the school was all but shut down for the summer. Walter wheeled up with a truck full of hockey sticks. I had to go and help him unload. He just lost track of time, he had the sticks, and Phyllis told him to get over here and drop them off before it was too late. I was the only one left here, and ready to go home. But how can you say no to Walter Gretzky?

I've only met Walter since his stroke. I live in the north end of Brantford near him, and I drive down his street every day, and he'll always wave at you. He's almost like a father to all Brantford's children. He's always running around doing stuff, and he's very hospitable.

There's a certain profile that comes from Walter Gretzky being associated with the school. The most famous hockey dad in the world! We enjoy the association. We encourage it. We count on his support, but it is really the fact that he enjoys the kids here that matters most. It's not just fundraising. To see Walter come in, it brightens everyone's day. It really does. He's a very positive man. As long as he wants to be a part of the school here, he's welcome.

Reaching out to others often means having to get up in front of people and speak, something I used to do only if I couldn't avoid it. The first time I was asked to speak after my stroke was for a CNIB fundraising event. I found that I actually liked to do it, and the audience response was really positive.

When Frank Rubini from the Heart and Stroke Foundation contacted me to find out if I'd be interested in getting involved as a spokesperson for that cause, it just seemed a natural thing for me to want to go out and spread the word about my experience of stroke and recovery. I've got so many stories to tell, and I love to make people laugh, as well as deliver a serious or inspirational message. I mean, funny things do happen to you when you are Wayne Gretzky's father.

For example, I went to Aurora one day to attend a birthday party for a fourteen-year-old boy. It was a skating party, and afterwards, the boy's father was hosting a lunch at which I was the guest speaker. I got there about an hour early, and as I was hanging around, waiting at the top of the arena, a lady came over and said, "Mr. Gretzky, could I get your autograph?" I said, "Sure," and reached into my pocket for one of the pads I usually carry. I didn't have one. I said, "I'm sorry, I haven't got anything to write on. Do you have something?"

"Yes, I have," she said.

I took out a blue magic marker and said, "Could I have it please?"

She pulled down her blouse.

"I beg your pardon?" I said.

"Would you mind?"

I was taken aback, to say the least. "What do you want me to write?"

She said, "What do you normally write?"

"What's your name?"

"Andrea."

I did my best, at arm's length, barely looking, to write "To Andrea, Best wishes, W. Gretzky." She was quite well-endowed— I could have written "Frank Mahovolich" on just the one side. After I was finished, she covered herself up and said, "Thank you very much, Mr. Gretzky. I'm going to show that to my boyfriend tonight." I couldn't believe it. I'll always remember that.

People's reactions can still amaze me sometimes. There was one occasion when Wayne and Janet were visiting in Brantford, and we all went to the mall. They wore ball caps and sunglasses, hoping that maybe they could have a quiet, private, normal time.

And I got mobbed, while they sat there watching from a bench! Finally, there were so many people, they figured they'd better help me out, and revealed themselves. I know it's a pain sometimes, but I really feel that if someone asks, you should give. Wayne gave a lot during his career, and he got a lot back, in terms of the respect and admiration of literally millions of people. Wayne understood that while his success was a real gift, it also came with responsibilities. The two of us have stayed up very late into the night on many occasions, just signing autographs on the cards, photos and other items that people send to us. I've seen people literally rip the shirt off Wayne's back, and I know why he has to travel now with security people most of the time. It's not the true fans he has a problem with, because they are respectful, but there are professional autograph and memento hunters who show up at every game and event. The same people, all the time. They're like stalkers. It kind of takes the fun out of it and spoils things for other fans, who really just want one special item to keep for themselves.

When I stand back from my life, it can seem like an odd way to live, always being recognized, having complete strangers come up to me and say hello, ask for an autograph, maybe tell me a story about meeting Wayne or seeing him play some time in the past, or just to thank me for having him in the first place. I'll be honest with you: Phyllis hates it! When we all started to be recognized in public, and someone would come up to her and ask, "Are you Wayne Gretzky's mother?" she'd sometimes actually say no, just to avoid having to be in the spotlight. She is gracious and will sign an autograph if asked, but that kind of situation has always made her feel awkward, and she would prefer not to have to deal with it. A long time ago, it just worked out that I'd be the front man for the family and she would be the one working behind the scenes. That suits her just fine.

Ask anyone who knows us, and they'll tell you that Phyllis is the glue that holds us all together. Honestly, I don't know what I'd have done without her through all the ups and downs of our lives over the years. I joke about the fact that she's the boss, but it's true. She's big-hearted and naturally down-to-earth, but she had to learn to be tough early on in Wayne's career, just to handle all the crazy things that can happen when your son is called the greatest hockey player who ever lived. Regardless of that turn of fate, she wanted to live as normal and as private a life as possible, which is understandable. She worked hard to maintain some order and sanity. Believe me, when you are this close to someone famous, you are bound to be approached by some questionable characters with questionable motives—good luck to them, in passing the Phyllis test. By now, she can spot the users a mile away. She's extremely protective of everyone in the family, but especially of Wayne and his privacy. If she wasn't, he would have a lot less of it than he does.

Traffic control alone in a household like ours can be a full-time job. In a town the size of Brantford, everybody knows where we live. For a very long time now, it has not been unusual for strangers to knock on our door, with any number of requests, some of which we can meet and some of which we can't. We try our best. I know Phyllis has been frustrated with me at times over the years, because I get out there and meet the public so much.

These days, there aren't too many places I go without being recognized. I was in St. John's, Newfoundland, one time, just walking up the street. A bus driver stopped his bus and came running across the street, with a big smile on his face, to shake my hand and say, "Hi Mr. Gretzky! I'd just like to say hello to you! You're a wonderful father. You've got a wonderful family." Then he ran back to the bus. He had a busload of people in there! Can you imagine?

FRANK RUBINI, HEART AND STROKE FOUNDATION: I took Walter, Ian and his kids along with my family to the Royal Ontario Museum in Toronto, and it was amazing how many people flocked over to Walter. The thing that really got me was when we were crossing University Avenue, people on the street were saying in the four-second interval when you pass, "Oh, that's Walter Gretzky!" Even on the Gardiner Expressway, in the summer, we've got the windows open, it's slow-going, a guy in the row over from us rolls his window down and yells over, "Hello, Mr. Gretzky, how ya doin?"

ROLY BYE: I once had to stop in to order something at the metal works outside of town, and a woman who worked there looked at my address, and when she saw it was Varadi Avenue, asked me, "Do you know Walter Gretzky?" I said, "Sure, we visit." She said, "You're kidding." I said, "No, we go for drives sometimes." She said, "No way!" I said, "Yes, it's true." Later, I took my wife Gloria, Ian and Walter out for a ride, and we stopped in there. I asked for the woman, and she came out and I said, "I've got my friend here." Well, honest to God, they pretty well shut the plant down. We got a tour of the whole place, and Walter shook everyone's hand. I remember another time, we went to a fish farm and they wanted his signature on a fish!

Now there are certain requests from fans that I'd never accommodate! I've travelled a lot with Ron Finucan, who works for the CNIB. Neither of us will forget the time we were at a special event, an air show, and one of the female skydivers, very beautiful, started getting extremely friendly with me. She was very forward, and very determined that I should become the father of her next child. She said this to me outright. She was someone who didn't like to take no for an answer, and as everyone knows, I am someone who has a hard time saying no. Ron laughs to this day, because when I finally managed to get away from her, I ran over to him and said, "Ron, we have to get out of here right now." He couldn't understand the hurry. I insisted. "We have to leave right this minute. That woman wants me to father her child, and Phyllis would be very upset with me if I did that." Ron and I hopped in a cab.

Parents come up to me, their babies in their arms, and ask me to touch them. Honestly, as though I am the Pope or something! I mean, I'm happy to pick up a baby, but I just don't understand that kind of request.

WAYNE: My father's so good with people. Everyone can relate to him. It's like they look up to him, and what he believes in and symbolizes, but at the same time, they recognize he's on the same plane as them. He does so many great things, and he's not motivated by money. I think that's why he's become

this Canadian icon. I swear, he could run for prime minister. I
believe there are lots of people who would vote for him!

Well, don't worry, I have no plans to pursue public office. But I take
what I do seriously and want to give value for the money people
donate to the causes I work for. Some would say too much value! I
remember being in North Battleford, Saskatchewan, at a luncheon to
raise funds for the CNIB. I was the guest speaker. I was up there at the
podium with my speech in front of me, talking away, when all of a
sudden, I see this hand come across and drop a piece of paper directly
in front of me. I finished my sentence, stopped for a second and
picked the paper up. It was a note from Ron Finucan: "Walter, cut it
short. These people have to get back to work." I crumpled it up,
threw it on the floor and kept talking. That's true, I'm not kidding.
Another time, Glen was travelling with me and promised to give me
a signal from the back of the room if I was running long—a finger
across his throat for "Cut it short!" Well, I was only two minutes into
the speech when I saw him signalling and I started to wrap it up. He
starts waving frantically for me to carry on—it turned out that his
throat had been itchy and he was just scratching it.

The lengths of my speeches vary. The last time I gave a talk, I
spoke for an hour and five minutes. That's too long. But on the
other hand, there can be such a thing as too short. When I go to a
function like a sports banquet, and they have six or eight speakers
who talk for five minutes, you might as well not let them get up.
Get one person to speak and be done with it!

One thing I quickly learned to do each time I made a speech
was to write out in big letters on a piece of paper where the heck

I was. I travel a lot, and with my memory lapses, I have been known to forget. Sometimes when I'm making a speech, my mind suddenly goes totally blank, and I forget what I just said. I forget everything. But I'll only be like that for a few seconds. Sometimes when I speak, I tell people, "If I stop for any reason, and I don't say anything for a few seconds, please bear with me. I don't have much of a memory," so they know what's going on. It doesn't bother me. There's nothing I can do about it.

Along with the funny things that have happened to me on the road, I've also seen some sadness. One day, a young boy came to our door and handed me a letter. I opened it and read, "Dear Mr. Gretzky, I want to play hockey this year, but our family has fallen on hard times. My father's out of work, my mother can't work, we have no money for registration. If you can help me, I would appreciate it, however if you can't, I still wish to thank you for reading the letter." He wrote the letter himself, but you could tell from the wording that someone told him what to say. I asked the boy, "Do you have a hockey stick?" He said no. So I went in the garage and got a stick. Any equipment? He said he had skates, but not much else. I said, "Okay, I'll be getting back in touch with you." Glen had been sitting on the couch in the living room through all this, and after the boy left, said, "Dad, his mother is across the road in a car." I looked out and there she was, sitting with her hand shielding her face, embarrassed but obviously determined to get someone to help her boy. I'll never forget that. I called a few organizations that have special funds for people in her situation and set things up. I called the boy at his home and got his mother on the line. I said, "It's Walter calling, just double-checking to see that your son got registered." And she said, "Yes, he did. Thank you very much." She was very nice, but I could tell she felt bad. I hope her boy enjoyed his season.

People know who I am and what I've been through and seem to feel comfortable telling me their problems. For reasons I don't fully understand, I often find myself called upon to offer sympathy and comfort to strangers. It's not unusual for people to confide in me about their tragedies and troubles—women in particular! I'm always willing to listen, and help if I can, but it takes me aback, because I'm not aware of what it is in me that they respond to. Not long ago, I was giving a luncheon speech in Brockville for the Heart and Stroke Foundation. After it was all over and people had left, I sat down at a table to finish my coffee and dessert. Then I saw two of the young waitresses coming towards me, one of them pushing the other in front of her, who seemed shy and reluctant. Of course I assumed she just wanted an autograph and got out my pen. But by the time the girl got to the table, she had burst into tears and was just sobbing. I really didn't know what to do. Her co-worker had to explain why she was so upset. Only a few weeks earlier, her brother, an avid hockey fan, had unaccountably dropped dead. He was only twenty-two, and no one knew what had caused his death. There had been absolutely no warning. Meeting me, the poor girl was just overcome with emotion—obviously, she wished her brother could have been there. When I went to sign my autograph to her, she asked that I make it out to her brother instead. I'm used to hearing these sad stories, but still, they always affect me, and some of them I can never forget.

It's the same kind of thing when I'm at home. The doorbell will ring. I'll say, "Can I help you?" And the person will say, "I've got a mother [or father, brother, sister, aunt, uncle, niece, nephew, son, daughter] who's only got two or three months to live. You weren't supposed to live the night, but look at you now. Can you come to the hospital with me?" The person will often start crying, right there on our doorstep, and say, "You'll be an inspiration to her. Maybe she'll live like you did. Please, can you come with me?" I get that so much, and I go.

Some friends of Roly's in Paris, Ontario, asked me to come see them once. The mother had had a stroke. Roly got hold of Ian and me, and asked if we would go. I said sure. Later, they told Roly that if it hadn't been for our visit, their mother wouldn't have made it. We were there for two hours, and I just tried to be positive and make them laugh a little, too. Now the lady is able to live by herself. I credit Ian with that. They had wanted to put her in a rehab centre. But Ian said to them, "You know, if you can get her one-to-one help, like Walter had, she'd be better off." They took Ian's advice, and she's very well today. Ian and I met the lady who became her therapist at a fundraising function at my grandson's school. Talking to her, and knowing what I know from my own experience of intensive individual therapy with Ian, I am convinced that this is what people need to help them recover. That and the love and support of family. I hope our health care system will move toward being able to accommodate one-to-one therapy as much as possible. Institutionalization should be a last resort.

I've learned over the years that it's not just older people who suffer strokes. There's one young lady I got to know here in town:

Crystal Walton. I think she's eighteen now. I met her after the doorbell rang one night and a couple of young people were standing on the doorstep telling me that their fifteen-year-old sister had had an aneurysm. Could I come to Hamilton and see her at the hospital there? Next day, I went to the hospital, the same one I had been in. Some of the nurses who had looked after me were there when I arrived. I was standing in the hallway, talking to them, when one of Crystal's family members came out of her room and said, "She's ready to see you." I walked in. She'd had a blood vessel burst in her brain and was totally paralyzed on her right side. They asked her, "Do you know who this is?" She said, "Of course, that's Walter." And for the first time in six weeks, she smiled with both sides of her mouth. Her face moved. Do you know how great it is to be part of a moment like that?

Her family had a homecoming celebration for her and asked if I'd come. Wayne was in Buffalo at the time, so I got an autographed picture for her, and he signed a get-well card. When the ambulance brought her home, I gave her the picture, the card and a couple of other things from Wayne. And then I gave her another little package, which was wrapped up, and I said, "Crystal, whenever you look at this, I want you to always remember the smile that you gave me the first time we met." She was in a wheelchair and could only use one hand. It was a digital watch that I gave her and she turned to me sideways and said, "Thanks, Walter." She smiled from ear to ear.

I go over there now to see her all the time. She lives a couple of blocks away. Crystal is up and walking, but she has to drag her foot. The police association in Cambridge bought her a computer to help her with her studies. She's a brilliant student.

Every year, at Christmastime, I take a couple of days and go along with a group of Ontario traffic police officers to some of the hospitals in the area, visiting the kids who are sick, giving out teddy bears, and little souvenirs and photographs of Wayne. And many generous people help us out—like Paul Arrowsmith at Kraft Canada, who every year gives us thousands of hockey cards for the kids. I really admire the officers who organize this and give of their time. There's a very special atmosphere in these places, very sad sometimes, but hopeful, too. Each time I visit, I have to take a deep breath and say to myself just before I go in, "Be brave now and maintain your composure."

Some of the kids have terminal illnesses, and they all have to be very strong and courageous in the face of their difficulties, as do their families. If I can help out at all with a visit, some words of encouragement, some little gifts, I'm happy to do it. I've got a good friend at Sears here in Brantford, Jerry Greenslade, who gets me dozens of digital watches every year, and when I go to the hospitals, I give them out to the older kids. Isn't that something, that every year my friend from Sears does that? They're not five-dollar watches either. They're nice watches. One time, we went into a room, and there was a girl there by herself, a fourteen-year-old. The OPP officer gave her a teddy bear, and I gave her a picture of Wayne, and a watch. She kept saying thank you, over and over and over. I was told later that she had terminal cancer. The girl had less than three months to live, yet she was so grateful because I gave her a watch.

KIM: At Mum and Dad's house, you know everybody goes downstairs to see all the awards and trophies that Dad has made into a shrine for the kids, but what he never shows them are the awards hanging in *his* office, such as the CNIB Arthur Napier Award, Brantford's Citizen of the Year, Honorary Big Brother, the Ontario Provincial Police Citation, Brantford General Hospital Volunteer Award, as well as a medal honouring his contribution to compatriots, community and country awarded by the Governor General to commemorate the 125th anniversary of Canada. And the dedication to my dad of a special Heart and Stroke Foundation Memorial Fund for Stroke.

For him, I know the awards are special, but he gets his real reward out of volunteering and helping people as much as he can, anyhow, anywhere.

But deep down, one event really meant a lot to him, and that was being inducted into the Brantford Walk of Fame at the same time as Alexander Graham Bell. When you think about it, here is a man who worked at Bell Canada for his whole life and now he's standing there on stage with relatives of Alexander Graham Bell.

My journey back to health and vitality was not an easy one, and I couldn't have done it alone. But maybe if you have made it all the way through this book, you have an idea now of what's possible for someone who survives an aneurysm. I accept my limitations, but if my loved ones had looked at the state I was in during those first hard years after my stroke and concluded, "This is it. This is how Walter will be now for the rest of his life," if they had given up on any kind of therapy for me, I would not be as well as I am today, speaking in public, helping kids and enjoying some time on the golf course.

I may be retired from my job at Bell, but I'm not retired from life! I can't even imagine wanting to have an idle "retirement."

Neither can Wayne. Back in 1999, when he decided to hang up his skates, I must admit, I was among those who really wished he wouldn't. I respected his decision and his right to make it, but a big part of me wanted to think he had a few more seasons in him yet. He knew my thoughts on the matter—I actively tried to talk him out of leaving—and that's why he kept his decision close to his chest until the last possible moment. Janet knew it was going to happen, and Phyllis too, but they kept it from me, knowing that there was a lot of media speculation around it, and that if anyone had asked me, I would have ended up spilling the beans. I'm just not someone who can tell a lie of any kind, and my social nature would have gotten the better of me eventually. Wayne told the two people he trusts most in this world, besides me—his wife and his mother—to make sure I didn't find out. He had other good reasons for not telling anyone, he told me later. He wanted as much as possible to keep the illusion in his mind that he would carry on playing. It was a psychological trick he played on himself to keep him from coasting through the final games or freezing with the thought that he was really playing his last NHL season. Even though it was.

Anyway, I guess I was always aware that the time was coming sooner rather than later. So it wasn't really a surprise when he phoned on a Thursday, and said, "Dad, come to my game in Ottawa." I knew then that that was going to be the last time my son played hockey on Canadian ice.

I don't recall much about the game itself, but afterwards, Bob Coyne and I drove back to Brantford. We stopped so many times along the way, I gave up counting. We had a cellphone in the car, and everyone somehow got wind of the number. That phone just kept ringing and ringing: "Hi, we're radio station so and so in some town you've never heard of, and since you guys are on the highway coming down from Ottawa, would you stop and give an interview?" We gave an interview to everyone who asked. I understood how important this event was to Canadians, and if they wanted my comments, I was prepared to provide them. Hockey fans deserved that, for sure. So many of them had come to equate their enjoyment of the game with watching Wayne play, and so many were almost in mourning or shock that his career on ice was finally coming to an end. Everyone wanted to talk to me about it.

And it was only a matter of a couple of days before Wayne's very last game at Madison Square Garden. He generously invited three of our close friends down there to join us for that: Butch, Eddie and Charlie. They were so touched.

WAYNE: I wanted my final games in Ottawa and New York to be a celebration, because some people were treating it as though it were a funeral, and I didn't want that. It was important for me to know that my dad and Janet especially, the two people in my life who would say that one of their biggest joys was watching me play hockey, were there that final night. We flew down to New York after the game in Ottawa. On the Saturday night, we all went out for dinner at a nice restaurant in Manhattan. It was a very special and private time for me, my family and our friends. My dad tried to talk me out of retiring right up to the last minute, but I was at peace with my decision. It absolutely felt right, and he knew that. But I think he is to this day a little confused as to why I decided to do it when I did. Sometimes he asks me if I'm going to come back, especially now that a few of the older players have recently done so. But my answer always was and always will be no. It's the right decision for me.

Sunday morning, just my dad and me, we took a cab—you don't drive in Manhattan!—and went down to the Garden early. It was important to me to share that final time alone with my dad. I just knew it was the right thing to do. Everything I have in my life has come to me because of hockey, because of my dad.

Was I sad watching my son skate around the ice for the very last time? I'm not sure I'd say that exactly. Maybe I didn't really let myself believe he'd never be playing hockey again. It was emotional. You could not be in that darkened arena, among all those thousands of fans, clapping and cheering on and on, as Wayne was down there waving goodbye, skating around and around on the ice by himself, and not feel something. Awe, really. I am his dad, but I feel just as amazed as anyone else when I think of what he has achieved over the years. It was one of those significant occasions that even someone with my kind of memory is never going to forget.

Well, maybe it's that crazy word "retirement" that I just keep stumbling over. When I consider the busy and varied life I lead today, I can't line it up with that concept. No reason why I should, in my opinion. I've got a lot of challenges to tackle, not to mention a lot of golf to play. Looking back on where I've been, I can only say I'm grateful, lucky to be alive, and raring to go wherever the next adventure takes me.

chapter eight

A LUCKY MAN

When I look back on my sixty-three years on this planet, I can honestly say that I feel like I've lived a thousand lifetimes. Not one, a thousand. All the different places I've been and things that have happened! Here, there, all over the world. It's wonderful to travel so much, have adventures with my good friends and meet such a wide variety of people—heads of state, native chiefs, Hollywood celebrities, sports legends, you name it—hear their stories and share some of mine. I hope to continue doing what I'm doing for a long time to come, as long as anyone asks me to share what I have learned over the years, before and since my stroke. And even though my direct involvement in hockey is scaled down now that I'm not coaching, it will always be the greatest sport around, in my opinion. I love to drop in at the local arenas, hang out and chat with whoever is there. Wayne may not be playing any more, but he's invited me down to training camp in Phoenix, and I'm keen to get a look at that. Keith's scouting for the Coyotes and living in Paris with his wife, Diana, and Brent is still playing for Fort Wayne in the United Hockey League and lives in Indiana with Nicole and the kids. (I still chew him out over his performance whenever the opportunity arises!)

PHYLLIS: He's happy as long as he's kept busy. I think people want to be around him because he likes to talk. He'll just walk up to strangers and start yakking away. He was not like that before. He would wave to the neighbours, but that was it. Now, he's out doing something for somebody all the time.

Maybe I should take more breaks—Phyllis sure thinks so—but all the travelling and socializing suits my restless spirit, no question. And with a family the size of ours, and with all the different activities everyone's got on the go, there's really never a dull moment at home either. It's great to have Glen around, who worked with his sister over the last couple of years to help me with this book. Kids, grandkids, dogs, cats and neighbours are coming and going all the time.

I like to go over to Phyllis's mother's house almost every day to keep her company and do any little chores she needs done. Since recovering from the stroke, I've also gotten into the habit of raking leaves and shovelling snow for some of our neighbours, ladies who've been widowed or who are unable to get out and do strenuous tasks. Wayne even bought me a snow blower last Christmas, so I can really do the job. My family thinks it's quite a joke, because let's just say that raking the leaves on my own lawn and shovelling the snow in my own driveway weren't exactly high priorities for me before the stroke.

I don't know exactly how or when my career as a neighbours' handyman got started. But I know there was a point when I understood that Ian and my family were concerned that I find ways to use my time, and I was eager myself to find things to do. I truly wanted to be useful. I had my energy back and didn't want to waste it. My neighbour Roly Bye recalls the time a few years ago, when I was becoming more mentally alert and starting to get out on my own more, and I went down the street to visit him. He was doing some work in the front yard. He'd had a backhoe come in and dig everything up and had a dump truck with topsoil sitting out there. Roly's chihuahua ran down the driveway and started yapping. Roly hollered at her from where he was in the backyard, wondering what the heck she was barking at. He came around to the front and saw it was me standing at the gate. I said, "Hey Roly, what are you doing with all this dirt?" He told me it was topsoil he had to spread. I said, "Where's a shovel? I'll give you a hand." He looked shocked and said, "Oh Wally, no, you're not going to shovel that. There's a dump truck full." But I said, "No, really, I've got some time." After all the things Roly had done for me, I felt it was the least I could do. But he said, "No, as a matter of fact,

I've got a professional coming in to do it." I thought he was just trying to discourage me. Finally I said to him, "Come on, you've been so good, can't I do anything?" He just kept saying no. Then we got out back and I saw his grass. I said, "Holy moly, Roly, when are you gonna cut your grass?" He said, "When I get around to it." So I said, "Well, where's your lawn mower? I'll cut your grass." He kept saying, "You don't need to cut the grass, Wally." But I insisted. I got the lawn mower and pulled the cord a couple of times, but it didn't start. Roly said, "It's not going to go, Wally. It's got no gas." But I knew there was gas in it, and I was determined to get it working. Poor Roly was late for an appointment and thought, "Oh brother, I'll never get out of here if I don't start the lawn mower for him." So he started it, and I mowed the yard. He shook his head. He just couldn't believe I wanted to cut his grass. He even took a picture. I was happy to do it, especially when I found out it was Roly and Gloria's wedding anniversary. Cutting his grass made me feel good. Here was something I could do for people, and I continue to do what I can for my neighbours.

I also attend church regularly when I'm at home. Our whole family feels comfortable there, because it's the same church we've been going to for years, and everyone knows us as ordinary parishioners, not famous people. There's no pretense there. Everyone needs a place like that to keep them grounded, and to keep in perspective what is truly important in life: family, community and nurturing the spiritual side of yourself. Ellen particularly enjoys it, because people at church are very accepting and kind and treat her with great respect.

Our church is special to us, and I like to help out with the charity work they do, their fundraising events and chores. Every year, we have Wayne Gretzky calendars made up, and I always donate lots of them to the church. I appear at charity auctions and drive shipments of donated toys and supplies to depots from where they're delivered to kids in Third World countries. There're so many things to do when you really start to get involved. Sounds crazy, but in a way, I find this kind of work the opposite of stressful. I've got a good friend, Betty Kelso, who works in the church office, and I love to duck in there unexpectedly through the back way now and then to chat with her. That's great downtime for me. I go during the week, when there's no one around and I can put up my feet and relax between errands and appointments. It's a wonderful change of pace from all the public appearances. And Betty spoils me. She knows I love orange suckers, and she always has a supply on hand just for me. No wonder I keep coming back!

I like to do things on the spur of the moment. Bob Coyne and I were at the church one time, and the minister was mailing out a big bunch of letters for all the parishioners. He was lamenting about the high cost of postage, so on an impulse, I said, "I'll take them." Bob and I drove all around the city and hand-delivered about 140 envelopes. I got a kick out of people's reactions. We would knock on the door, and people would come and say, "Oh, it's Walter Gretzky!" I would shake their hands, give them their letter and say, "I'm just delivering this for the church." We had so much fun, we did it twice. Of course, we could have simply gone to the post office and paid for the postage ourselves, because the money we put out in gas far exceeded the cost of stamps! But you know, the people enjoyed it, which made it worth doing. I've volunteered to do it whenever they want. Now I gather that word has spread through the church that Walter delivers letters.

But I'm not all work and no play, despite what some people might tell you. The other place where you'll often find me when I'm not on the road, is the golf course. I'm always itching to get out there once the snow has melted, and will golf right through until the ground freezes up again. On one level, it's good fun and exercise—as I've said, I like to keep moving. But I think maybe there's more to it than that; it has helped in my recovery by building up my confidence. I started out as a non-golfer, and my friends still tell me I've got the craziest swing known to mankind. But it works for me. I know some people suspect me of lying about my scores, but this is where a memory problem comes in handy: I can always claim that I simply forgot! The course is a place for me to kid around with the guys, and I'm sure Phyllis enjoys having me out of her hair on those long summer days. I like to tell my stories in the clubhouse, and in a way, it's a testing ground for my speeches. There are always groups of people there willing to listen, and I'll gauge from their reaction whether a story is one that will work for an audience. I'm always trying to perfect my speaking style and find new material that will be entertaining to a crowd.

I've met some remarkable people in my travels and made some great friends wherever I've gone, but sometimes you don't even have to leave your street to find a special friend in this world. Take Daniel Eickmeier. I met him on Halloween night, about seven years ago. Daniel was eight years old at the time. I didn't know his family; they were new to the street. They had moved to Brantford from Windsor, so that Daniel could attend the W. Ross Macdonald School, where they have terrific programs for kids like him— programs you can't find anywhere else. As well as being visually impaired, he has some motor problems that make walking difficult for him, so his mother took him out trick-or-treating separately from her other two kids.

That first Halloween, Daniel stood at our door in his costume and started asking me questions about myself. He knew something had happened to me, but he wasn't sure what it was. At one point— I'll never forget his tone of voice or how he worded it, so thoughtful and mature for a boy of only eight—he said, "Well, Mr. Gretzky, how long was it after your medical mishap that you were able to speak to your friends and your family?" That's when I figured out what he was doing. He wasn't asking about me; he was asking about his dad. We were aware, you see, that Daniel's father, who was only in his early forties, had recently had a stroke and couldn't yet talk. Daniel was obviously wondering when his dad was going to talk again. Talking with his dad was crucial to Daniel, because he can't see.

I was deeply touched by this intelligent, curious and brave little boy, and decided to get to know Daniel and his family better. Now he and I are great buddies. I like to bring him souvenirs from wherever I've travelled. Sometimes, too, I'll go down and visit late at night, when Daniel and the other kids are in bed, just to have a chat and cup of tea with his mum and dad, who are great people. I think at first, they wondered who the heck was knocking on their door that late. But now, they know it's just me, and we enjoy our conversations. I just like to see how they are doing, because although they are very strong people who handle their difficulties beautifully, I know they've got a lot on their shoulders, and want them to know I am there for them.

Daniel's met Wayne, too, and is a great fan. We've even gone golfing together, and he is a key part of our annual fundraising tournament for the CNIB. There's a nice painted portrait of Daniel and me out on the golf course, right in the foyer of the W. Ross Macdonald School. They're as proud of him there as I am. We talk about all kinds of things. He's a teenager now, and I'm sure he has a very bright future ahead of him, because he's so smart. He's into ham radio and communicates with people all over the world.

I love to do special things for him whenever I can. There's one time I'll always remember. Back in 1997, on a beautiful September day, I decided to take Daniel to a Blue Jays game. He is their number one fan. He listens to every game on his radio headset. Tom and Jerry, the voices of the Jays, are special to him. He knows them like friends, because they're in his head all the time. So I called Bob Coyne, who knows Daniel from the school, and told him, "I'd love to take him down to the game. You know a bit more about travelling with blind kids than I do. Would you come with us?" Bob said sure, and away we went to the game in Toronto.

Now, Robbie Alomar, one of Daniel's favourite players, had been traded to the Baltimore Orioles, and was coming to play against the Jays that night. So I phoned Tom Bitove, Wayne's partner in the restaurant, which is right near the SkyDome and where they know Robbie, and they made arrangements for Daniel to meet him. I wanted it to be a big surprise. We had an early supper at the restaurant (Tom and all the staff there always treat us so well they make us feel like *we* own the place) and then went over to SkyDome. It was late afternoon when we got there, batting practice time. We looked around and sure enough, there were the restaurant people standing with Robbie. We didn't say a word to Daniel as they ushered us out onto the field, and we walked right up to Alomar. He leaned down and said, "Hi, Daniel." Well, Daniel knows the players' voices, and his face just lit up. "Robbie Alomar!" he said. You could see what a thrill it was for him. Robbie talked to Daniel and gave him an equipment bag filled with baseballs, caps, pins and other baseball paraphernalia, items signed by all of the Baltimore Orioles. Then, Robbie leaned down and said to him, "Daniel, you know what I'm gonna do for you tonight? I am going to hit a home run, especially for you." I was thinking, "Uh-oh, what if he doesn't!" But with that, he gave Daniel a rub on the top of his head and said, "I've got to go to batting practice now. I'll see you later."

At that moment, Brian Williams from CBC Sports, who was there to cover the game, saw me, came right over and said, "Walter Gretzky, how are you? What are you doing here?" I said, "I brought my friend Daniel to meet Robbie Alomar." Brian saw that Daniel was blind and said, "I'll bet you'd also like to meet Tom and Jerry. I can take you up there right now." So we left the field and took a special elevator up to the broadcasting booth. Tom and Jerry let Daniel recite the lineup that night, and then they showed him how they do their special effects. They let him play with all the gizmos and gadgets in the broadcasting booth, and he had a wonderful time. As we were leaving, one of them asked us,

"Where are you guys sitting?" And I said, "Exactly behind home plate, front row." And he said, "Okay, we're going to alert the TV crew, and they're going to put you on the big screen several times tonight, and we want to mention Daniel's name in the broadcast." We left the booth and took our seats.

It was a regular baseball game, nothing special. In the seventh inning, Robbie came to the plate. He'd been up two or three times prior to that and had got a single twice, I think, but no home run. Here in the seventh inning, he was up again, and he faced the pitcher, who slid the ball down, and bang, Robbie knocked it right out of the park. The interesting thing to note here is that at that particular time in Robbie Alomar's career, he was being ostracized by fans for a spitting incident with an umpire. And so he was not exactly popular in Toronto. But the crowd around us had heard that Robbie Alomar was going to hit a home run for Daniel, and when that happened, there was a standing ovation just in the little zone where we were sitting. After he finished running the bases, he came across home plate and ran back to that rope-type mesh that was between us and the playing field. He reached through, grabbed Daniel by the hand and said, "Daniel, that was for you."

BOB COYNE: I thought I was gonna die, right there on the spot. No one other than Walter Gretzky could have orchestrated that. I certainly couldn't have produced an evening like that for a little boy. No way. Not many of us could. But Walter, because of who he is, has access to an awful lot. There are many other Canadians who have as much standing as

Walter, but they don't use it the way he does. Walter probably didn't even want to go to the ball game himself. But there he was that evening, to provide a thrill of a lifetime for a kid, and he did it.

I've got another special friend, Jesse, who is also visually impaired and a former student of the W. Ross Macdonald School. He's in his twenties now, but our whole family got to know him well while he was at the school. A few years ago, we had one fabulous time together, thanks to Wayne and my (second) favourite game, golf.

Every year, at the CNIB golf tournament, we have a charity auction of various prizes. Gino Reda, the sportscaster, always moderates. He is a wonderful guy, a wholehearted participant in the event, who has been very generous with his time and efforts over the years. One of the items up for auction that particular year was an all-expenses-paid vacation for four to St. Andrews Links in Scotland. Now, golf courses don't get any better than that, and everyone knew it was a real plum of a package and deserved some good bids. But bidding was slow. Wayne was there, of course, and thought, "What the heck, I'll buy up this one." He wanted to send me, Gino, Ron Finucan and Jesse for one special week of golfing we'd never forget.

It was funny, because after the announcement that Wayne had bought the package for the four of us, Gino's young son ran over to his dad, who was busy with something else, and shouted "Dad, Dad, Wayne Gretzky is sending you over to golf in Scotland!" Gino thought his son had simply gotten mixed up, and said to him, "No, no, that's not happening." When he finally was told that it was definitely happening, he just couldn't believe it.

That was one memorable vacation for all of us, I'll tell you. Especially for Jesse, because he fulfilled two big dreams on that trip. He had never been on an airplane, and he'd never been to the ocean. And he was always saying that among all the things he wanted to do in his life, flying in a plane and going to the ocean were right up there on his "must do" list.

St. Andrews itself is spectacular, right on the North Sea. Every day, we'd drive to the course along those narrow, windy roads, and I particularly enjoyed the sight of the sheep and their lambs scampering around on the green hillsides. It was quite magical. Our accommodations were incredible, as were our meals, although there was one dinner that didn't sit well with me, and Gino and Ron don't let me forget it. I was so taken with the peaceful sight of all the lambs on the hillsides. But one evening, unbeknownst to me, we were served lamb. Naturally, it's a specialty in the fine restaurants there, but I wasn't clued in to that. I began my meal and then asked, "What's this we're eating, anyway?" When someone said "lamb," I was stunned. I didn't want to be rude, but I really could not bring myself to eat it. I just put down my knife and fork and wouldn't eat any more, claiming I wasn't hungry. But Gino and Ron knew I was thinking about all those little lambs I'd seen, and asked the chef to prepare something else for me to eat.

Ron and Gino had died and gone to golf heaven, of course, and I was having a pretty good time there, too. But in the first couple of days, my chief concern wasn't playing golf; it was making sure that Jesse got the chance to realize his second dream. It was fine to be near the sea, but from the course, all he could really experience was the sound of it.

My buddies tease me about that trip to this day. I really would not let up until I had figured out a way to get Jesse near the water. At one end of the course there were some rocks along an incline to the shore, very rugged, but if you went gingerly you could walk along until you got down to the sea. So one morning, I just said, "Come on Jesse, let's go." Ron and Gino wondered how the heck we were going to do it, and followed behind us, as I led Jesse along by the hand. They were worried that we were going to fall in, since I can sometimes list to one side and Jesse couldn't see his footing. It was fairly precarious and slippery, but I was determined. And in the end, we did it. When we finally got down to the sea, I made sure Jesse got to dip his hand in the water, to get a real sense of where he was. I said, "Here we are, Jesse. Now you can really say you've been to the ocean." It was a special moment for Jesse and for all of us, I think.

When you go to the W. Ross Macdonald School, you'll see its motto on the wall: The Impossible Is Only The Untried. It dates back to the late 1800s, but no one knows who wrote it. I think it is an excellent motto for anyone to have, whatever their capabilities. I believe we all have to challenge ourselves every day to be our best. Sometimes, what seems impossible really is only something that you haven't tried. No one who saw me back in the days after my stroke would have believed I'd be here today, offering you these thoughts, sharing with you a few glimpses of my life. Every day, it seems, something new happens that gives me a fresh perspective on life, and I have to say I'm happy to be alive.

My involvement as a spokesperson for the Heart and Stroke Foundation has also brought me many wonderful moments, just connecting and relating with people who are going through similar problems as mine.

FRANK RUBINI: I remember one woman in particular from Trenton who wrote the Heart and Stroke Foundation to thank us for recruiting Walter as our stroke spokesperson. She had been going about her usual day, driving somewhere, when she started to feel uncomfortable. She had no history of heart disease or stroke in her family, but what she was feeling reminded her of the signs and symptoms of stroke described in a front-page article in her local newspaper. Only days before, Walter and I had been near her town as part of a national media tour for the Foundation. A journalist from the local paper covered the story and listed the signs and symptoms of stroke in the article.

Because of the information she learned from that article, she decided to exit the highway and seek help. She pulled into a strip mall and parked her car in front of her favourite butcher shop. As soon as she opened the car door and went to get out, she collapsed, and a person from the shop ran out to help. She was rushed to hospital and treated with a new time-sensitive drug treatment for ischemic strokes (caused by a blockage in a blood vessel in the brain) and made a near-perfect recovery.

I found out later that this woman was only forty-seven years old, with four children. Walter and I still talk about how different that woman's life would have been if Walter hadn't made that speech in Kingston.

Walter never wants to admit that he has such an impact on people's lives, but he does. I travel with him and I witness the effect he has on people and how they listen so intently to every word he says. I have to admit that I live my life differently as a result of knowing Walter, his family and their philosophy of life.

As far as I'm concerned, no one should ever have to feel that they are alone in their struggle toward recovery. When that feeling of isolation sets in, it's easy to give up, and that's the last thing you should do. In reaching out and touching people, giving them some hope, I enjoy my role immensely. Helping others to hang in there and figure out how to get over all the obstacles, which I know intimately because I've had to overcome them myself, is what it's all about, in my opinion.

As part of the campaign to raise public awareness about stroke and the work of the foundation, we shot a TV advertisement last winter at the farmhouse, outside, down by the river. It made sense to do it there. After all these years, it's still the place that I call home, the place to which I have the deepest spiritual connection, to my parents and to my past. Of all the places I've been in the world, this is still where I feel most myself and most at peace.

The people producing the ad debated whether they should give me a script or not, and in the end, they figured they'd just let me say whatever I wanted. That seemed more natural and was fine by me. I prefer to just go with the flow. The guy with the camera stood across the river, aimed it at me and shouted, "Just say whatever comes to mind!"

At first, I thought, "What the heck am I gonna say?" I was standing there on the riverbank, holding the hand of my grandson Nathan, and I just looked out at the river and looked back at him.

And then I did say what came to my mind: "To think that when I was his age, I used to come down to this very spot on the river and fish, swim and play. And here I am today, standing in the very same spot with our grandson."

I may not have the best memory around, but I can say one thing: I know how to appreciate what's happening in the present. I can live joyfully in the moment better than I ever did before my medical crisis. And at moments like that one, I feel as though my life truly has come full circle. It's a blessing that fills me with happiness and gratitude.

When Phyllis and I pull up the driveway at the farm, where we hold all our family get-togethers, we walk past the door to the cellar where I dropped that paintbrush ten years ago. Inside the house, surrounded by Phyllis and our children—and our grandchildren, who come running up to me saying, "Grandpa, will you please take us fishing?"—I realize I truly am a lucky man.

AFTERWORD

I want to put my national spokesperson hat on here, and tell you
a few crucial things about stroke. Most strokes are caused by a
blood clot blocking the blood flow to the brain. They're sort of
like heart attacks, but in the brain (doctors call this an ischemic
stroke). But mine was different, and much less common. My
stroke was caused by the rupture of a blood vessel in my brain. It
turns out that one of my blood vessels had a weak spot, which
caused it to bulge out like a balloon. This weak spot (doctors call
it an *aneurysm*) could have been something I was born with, or

might have been caused by my accident in those early days working for Bell Canada. No one will ever really know.

What I do know is that in 1991, that weak spot gave way. The effect was like a tire blowing when you're driving down the road—big trouble! I'd had headaches all my life but when my blood vessel burst, I had a crushing headache like nothing I've ever had before. It took everything in me to make it upstairs to the kitchen at the farm. I had double vision. I could hardly walk or talk.

The good news is that someone was there who recognized the signs of stroke—and reacted right away. She could see that I was in serious trouble and got me to the closest hospital in no time flat. Eventually, I was sent to Hamilton for brain surgery, but I wouldn't have made it if someone hadn't been there, recognized what was wrong and immediately got me to a hospital.

Doctors call the type of stroke I had a *subarachnoid hemorrhage*. That's their term for uncontrolled bleeding on the surface of the brain, between the brain and the skull. The bleeding came from that burst vessel. To stop the bleeding, doctors put a clip (sort of like a clothes pin) on the blood vessel. Doctors say the clip should last for as long as I will. So I'm lucky, in that I don't have to worry about the stroke coming back. Also, because I had a stroke caused by bleeding, I had to have a tube called a shunt implanted to drain fluid from my brain. Most stroke patients don't need those sorts of things, but I guess I'm in a sort of special class. Only about 10 per cent of strokes are subarachnoid hemorrhages.

But no matter what kind of stroke you have, the effect is basically the same—there is damage to the brain. The brain controls everything you say, do, think and remember, so a stroke can affect a lot of different things. After a stroke, some people may be paralyzed on one side; others might have trouble talking or understanding speech. Because the brain is so complicated, a stroke can even affect your personality, how you act, or how you see or understand things. In my case, because of where the bleeding happened, the main thing that's been affected is my memory.

I'm told that out of every four people who have a stroke, one will die, one will recover fully, one will recover but not completely and one will be left severely disabled. So I count myself as one of the lucky ones. With the help of my family, doctors and therapists, I've made a great recovery. If it wasn't for my memory problems, most people would never know that I've had a stroke. Now, I'm working with the Heart and Stroke Foundation to help other people learn the warning signs of stroke and the need to get to the hospital right away. I feel really fortunate that the Foundation has given me the chance to use my experience to help other people. It's my chance to keep reminding people that I'm alive today because someone knew the warning signs of stroke. I hope that someday everyone will know them. Here they are:

WARNING SIGNS OF A STROKE

Weakness
Sudden weakness, numbness or tingling in the face, arm or leg

Trouble Speaking
Sudden temporary loss of speech or trouble understanding speech

Vision Problems

Sudden loss of vision, particularly in one eye, or double vision

Headache

Sudden, severe and unusual headache

Dizziness

Sudden loss of balance, especially with any of the above signs

If you or someone you know is having any of these signs, call 911 or your local emergency number immediately.

For more information on stroke, please contact your local Heart and Stroke Foundation office.